THE ULTIMATE GUIDE TO PHYSICIAN ASSOCIATE OSCEs

THE ULTIMATE GUIDE TO PHYSICIAN ASSOCIATE OSCEs

AMEENA AZAD

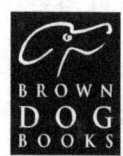

BROWN DOG BOOKS

First published 2021

Copyright © Ameena Azad 2021

The right of Ameena Azad to be identified as the author of this work has been asserted in accordance with the Copyright, Designs & Patents Act 1988.

All rights reserved. No part of this book may be reproduced, stored in a retrieval system, or transmitted in any form or by any means, electronic, electrostatic, magnetic tape, mechanical, photocopying, recording or otherwise, without the written permission of the copyright holder.

Although the author and publisher have made every effort to ensure that the information in this book was correct at press time, the author and publisher do not assume and hereby disclaim any liability to any party for any loss, damage, or disruption caused by errors or omissions, whether such errors or omissions result from negligence, accident, or any other cause.

Published under licence by Brown Dog Books and The Self-Publishing Partnership Ltd, 10b Greenway Farm, Bath Rd, Wick, nr. Bath BS30 5RL

www.selfpublishingpartnership.co.uk

ISBN printed book: 978-1-83952-309-0
ISBN e-book: 978-1-83952-311-3

Internal design by Mac Style

Printed and bound in the UK

This book is printed on FSC certified paper

Practice OSCE stations with these checklists with tips and guidance throughout. This book is the first OSCE book tailored directly to Physician Associate (PA) OSCE exams. This book will prepare you for your university and national OSCE exams at a high standard.

About the Author

I am a qualified Physician Associate, working in general practice. Although having good medical knowledge is crucial to make a good and safe clinician, a lot of it is down to communication. This book will allow you to practise against these checklists on your own or with family/friends, which will mean you will get sleek and confident with whatever the station throws at you. I passed all my university OSCE exams with very high averages and I passed all 14 stations at the OSCE nationals first time round, also with very high averages. I wanted to create a realistic guide for Physician Associate OSCEs, directly tailored to PA students. As a student, there were no resources tailored directly to us, hence the desire for wanting to write this book and help to grow our PA community. I have included tricks and tips that I learnt from my experiences and from what my peers have also told me.

This book will be broken down in accordance with the OSCE blueprint covering common and most likely presentations that may come up as an OSCE station. In accordance with the OSCE blueprint on the Faculty of Physician Associate (FPA) page, this book will try to follow a checklist format and practice stations according to the weighting on the blueprint:

- Consultation skills
- Examination skills
- Procedural skills
- Emergency management

Contents

Consultations   1
1. Focused diagnostic history   1
2. Information giving   12
3. Motivational interviewing (e.g. smoking cessation)   15
4. Breaking bad news   18
5. Dealing with conflict   21
6. Telephone communication (peer to peer handover – SBAR)   22

Examination skills   24
1. Vital signs (temperature, pulse rate, respiratory rate, saturation monitoring and blood pressure) including EWS/MEWS type score calculation   24
2. Nutrition e.g. calculating BMI   26
3. Lumps and bumps (describe and diagnose)   26
4. Hand examination   29
5. Spine cervical examination   31
6. Hip examination   34
7. Knee examination   37
8. Shoulder examination   39
9. Rashes and skin disorders   41
10. Lymphoreticular system   43
11. Cardiovascular examination   45
12. Peripheral vascular examination   49
13. Respiratory examination   52
14. Diabetic foot examination   55
15. Neurological eye examination (inc ophthalmoscopy)   58
16. Cranial nerve exam   62
17. Peripheral nervous system – upper limb   67
18. Peripheral nervous system – lower limb   71
19. Cerebellar examination   75
20. ENT– auroscopy   78
21. Gastrointestinal examination   80
22. Rectal examination   83
23. Hernia examination   85

24. Pregnant abdomen — 87
25. Breast examination — 88
26. Mental state examination — 90
27. Verification of death (not certification, checking for signs of life) — 94

Procedural skills — 95
1. Urinalysis and interpretation — 95
2. IM injection — 96
3. SC injection — 98
4. Venepuncture — 100
5. Performing an ECG — 102
6. Checking peak flow — 104
7. Arterial blood gas sampling — 105
8. Catheterisation – FEMALE — 107
9. Catheterisation – MALE — 110
10. Cannulation — 114
11. Suturing — 116
12. Speculum — 118
13. Nasogastric tube insertion and position checking — 121
14. Wound care and dressings — 123
15. Obtaining ENT and skin swabs — 123

Emergency management — 124
1. BLS — 124
2. Immediate Life Support (airway management and simple arrhythmia recognition and management) — 125
3. Choking — 126
4. ABCDE approach — 127
5. Oxygen therapy — 130
6. Initial seizure management — 131
7. Recognition and reversal of poisoning e.g. opiates — 132
8. Manage electrolyte disturbances e.g. hyperglycaemia, hypoglycaemia — 132
9. Fluid resuscitation in shock e.g. blood loss — 135
10. Sepsis management — 135
11. 1st aid – nose bleed — 137

Reference List — 139

* WASH AND GEL HANDS FOR ALL STATIONS *

1
Consultations

FOCUSED DIAGNOSTIC HISTORY

Case Scenario 1

In A&E a gentleman presents with chest pain. Your supervising registrar asks you to take a focused history and then to discuss a management plan. Please only take a history, no examination is required. (TIP: the word 'focused'; always read the case properly before entering the station and spot the key words)

1 ICE – Introduction, Consent and Exposure (not needed in this scenario)

Introduce yourself: full name and your role

Confirm patient identity (name and date of birth)

Ask for consent: 'Is it okay if I take a history from you?'

As it's a focused history, instead of starting with an open question, you can say, 'I understand you have come in with chest pain, can you please tell me more about it?'

2 History of Presenting Complaint

Pain – SOCRATES (site, onset, character, radiation, associated symptoms, timing, exacerbating and relieving factors such as change in position or medication and severity scale)

Associated cardiovascular symptoms can include: palpitations, shortness of breath, dizziness, orthopnoea, paroxysmal nocturnal dyspnoea (PND), ankle swelling – (NB if a patient is describing a classic myocardial infarction (MI) you may not need to ask about orthopnoea at this point)

Classic MI symptoms: central crushing and heavy chest pain, or more to the left, radiating down the arm, shoulders, back and into the jaw, sweating, clammy, light headedness/dizziness, shortness of breath, palpitation, nausea/vomiting and abdominal pain

Associated respiratory symptoms can include: shortness of breath, cough–productive? Haemoptysis? Wheezing, calf pain or swelling, pleuritic pain

Associated gastrointestinal symptoms can include: dyspepsia, abdominal pain, nausea and vomiting, pain worse on lying, relieved by leaning forward

Red flags and systemic symptoms: weight loss, night sweats, fevers and pain elsewhere

Quick review of a general system review (if appropriate):

MSK: joint/muscle/bone pain, stiffness, swelling

Neurology: vision changes, headaches, sensory changes, loss of consciousness (LOC) or convulsions

GI: change in bowel habits, abdominal pain, ALARMS (anaemia, loss of weight, anorexia, recent changes, melaena and dysphagia)

Urology: polyuria, dysuria, urgency, haematuria, abdominal pain

3 Past Medical History

Explore their past medical history so you can ask, 'Do you have any diagnosed medical conditions, such as high blood pressure, diabetes etc.?' Remember THREAD (thyroid, hypertension, rheumatoid arthritis, epilepsy, asthma and diabetes) and remember to refrain from using medical jargon if possible. Ask if they have had any previous MIs or cardiovascular-related issues in the past.

4 Drug History

It is ideal to ask about the drug history after asking about the past medical history. If they state they have hypertension, you can question them about their ACEi/ARB/CCB medication. In a cardiovascular setting ask specifically about aspirin, statins etc. (NB ask about dosage, route, how many times a day)

Explore any allergies at this point.

5 Family History

Explore any family history here: 'Can I ask about any medical illnesses that run in your family?' Give examples, such as 'diabetes, high blood pressure, high cholesterol, MIs/heart disease particularly if under 50, heart failure, DVT/PEs. (NB if they say e.g. their mother has passed away after a heart attack, remember to acknowledge that and show empathy.)

6 Social History

Explore: Smoking – pack years, alcohol intake, use of any recreational drugs, lifestyle, diet, any physical fitness, occupation, any issues at home/stress-related?

7 Travel History

In a cardiovascular history long-haul flights are relevant due to risks of DVT/PE.

In a respiratory/infection history– possible chance of infection.

Additional Marks

This will depend on how you communicate the station; did you show empathy, did you listen actively and acknowledge? The use of both open and closed questions is important. Be sure to explore the 2nd ICE – Ideas, Concerns and Expectations – 'Any thoughts on what this could be?' 'Are you concerned about anything in particular?'

Summarise and then ensure that you have met the patient's expectations. 'This is the plan. Are you happy with what we have discussed/was this what you were expecting?'

If you are expected to turn to the examiner or discuss with the patient and explain a diagnosis or initial investigations or discuss a management plan, always give a quick summary and always offer differential diagnoses, e.g. of initial management: if this patient was presenting with typical MI symptoms, discuss the use of MONAC.

M   Morphine
O   Oxygen
N   Nitrates
A   Aspirin
C   Clopidogrel

If they ask for investigations, first state that you will carry out a full examination, clinical observation such as pulse rate, respiratory rate, etc. and then use BOXES:

B   Bloods (FBC, U&Es, Cardiac markers – Troponin)
O   Orifice testing – Sputum, urine, stool
X   X-ray (Chest x-ray)
E   ECG
S   Special test i.e. MRI/CT

Remember avoid using jargon and finally, if you are sending this patient home, remember always SAFETY NET.

FOCUSED DIAGNOSTIC HISTORY

Case Scenario 2

A 32-year-old female presents with headache at the GP surgery that you work in. Take a focused history only and discuss your possible diagnosis.

1 ICE – Introduction, Consent and Exposure (not needed in this scenario)

Introduce yourself: full name and your role

Confirm patient identity (name and date of birth)

Ask for consent: 'Is it okay if I take a history from you?' 'I understand you have been suffering with headaches, can you please tell me more about it?' (Remember FOCUSED)

2 History of Presenting Complaint

Pain – SOCRATES (site, onset, character, radiation, associated symptoms, timing, exacerbating and relieving factors such as change in position or medication and severity scale)

Site: Unilateral, bilateral, timing: different times of the day

Remember your red flags for headaches: Raised intracranial pressure (ICP) (projectile vomiting, LOC, waking you up from sleep, if sneezing, coughing, bending or lying down makes it worse). Meningitis (rash, neck stiffness, photophobia). Stroke/transient ischaemic attack (TIA)/Temporal arteritis (vision disturbance, weakness, temporal tenderness, slurred speech)

Red flags and systemic symptoms: weight loss, night sweats, fevers and pain elsewhere

Quick review of a general system review (if appropriate):

MSK: joint/muscle/bone pain, stiffness, swelling

Urology: polyuria, dysuria, urgency, haematuria, abdominal pain

3 Past Medical History

Explore their past medical history so you can ask 'Do you have any diagnosed medical conditions, such as migraines, cluster headaches, any history of TIA or strokes?' Remember THREAD (thyroid, hypertension, rheumatoid arthritis, epilepsy, asthma and diabetes) and remember to refrain from using medical jargon if possible.

4 Drug History

It is ideal to ask about the drug history after asking about the past medical history. Always ask about anticoagulation/ anti-platelets in headaches, especially if head injury is involved. New onset migraine? Are they on a combined oral contraceptive pill (COCP)? (There is a link between migraines and COCP.) (NB ask about dosage, route, how many times a day.)

Explore any allergies at this point.

5 Family History

Explore any family history here: 'Can I ask about any medical illnesses that run in your family?' Give examples, such as 'migraines, malignancies, strokes/TIAs, or intracranial bleeds) (NB if they say e.g. their mother has passed away to a stroke, remember to acknowledge that and show empathy.)

6 Social History

Explore: smoking – pack years, alcohol intake, use of any recreational drugs, lifestyle, diet, any physical fitness, occupation, any issues at home/stress-related?

7 Travel History

Ask specifically about any recent travel abroad. Possible infection?

Additional Marks

This will depend on how you communicate the station: did you show empathy, did you listen actively and acknowledge? The use of both open and closed questions is important. Be sure to explore the 2nd ICE – Ideas, Concerns and Expectations – 'Any thoughts on what this could be?' 'Are you concerned about anything in particular?'

Summarise and then ensure that you have met the patient's expectations. 'This is the plan. Are you happy with what we have discussed/was this what you were expecting?'

Possible diagnosis: will depend on patient's presentation. It is very important to cover all headache differentials in depth such as migraines (different types), cluster headaches, tension headaches and the headaches that cause red flag symptoms. Remember SAFETY NET.

FOCUSED DIAGNOSTIC HISTORY

Case Scenario 3

A 26-year-old female comes to see you at your practice. She is complaining of abnormal discharge. Take a history only and discuss your management plan with the patient.

1 ICE – Introduction, Consent and Exposure (not needed in this scenario)

Introduce yourself: full name and your role

Confirm patient identity (name and date of birth)

Ask for consent: 'Is it okay if I take a history from you?'

2 History of Presenting Complaint

If there is pain use SOCRATES (site, onset, character, radiation, associated symptoms, timing, exacerbating and relieving factors such change in position or medication and severity scale)

Discharge? Explore: always start with checking and clarifying where the discharge is coming from (DO NOT ASSUME). Onset, duration, how did it start, has it changed during that time, colour, odour and consistency

In all gynaecological histories, remember MOSC (NB if they are not sexually active, only M should be used, therefore always ask if they are sexually active first)

M   Menstrual history: last monthly period (LMP), length of cycles, menorrhagia, dysmenorrhoea. Any bleeding out of cycle (intermenstrual bleed, post-coital bleed)
O   Obstetrics history: pregnancies, including miscarriages, terminations and stillbirths (be sensitive at this point)
S   Sexual history: explore practices, one or more partners, previous history of sexually transmitted infection
C   Contraception: which type, if using any

If sexually active, ensure to ask about whether they are up to date with their cervical smears. When was your last smear? Was everything normal? Smears are usually every 3 years for age ranges 25–64

Explore any possible gynaecological red flags, post-menopausal bleeding, bleeding during pregnancies, severe lower abdominal pains and bleeding

Red flags and systemic symptoms: weight loss, night sweats, fevers and pain elsewhere

Quick review of a general system review (if appropriate)

3 Past Medical History

Explore their past medical history so you can ask, 'Do you have any diagnosed medical conditions, such as polycystic ovaries, fibroids, endometriosis? Any previous history of ectopic pregnancies, have you previously lost any pregnancies?'

4 Drug History

It is ideal to ask about the drug history after asking about the past medical history. Always ask about anticoagulation/anti-platelets if bleeding is involved. (NB ask about dosage, route, how many times a day)

Explore any allergies at this point.

5 Family History

Explore any family history here: 'Can I ask about any medical illnesses that run in your family?' Give examples, such as cervical or endometrial cancer, fibroids or any bleeding disorders.

6 Social History

Explore: Smoking – pack years, alcohol intake, use of any recreational drugs, lifestyle, diet, any physical fitness, occupation, any issues at home/stress-related (if relevant)?

7 Travel History

Ask specifically about any recent travel abroad, had intercourse with anybody abroad. Possible sexually transmitted infection?

Additional Marks

This will depend on how you communicate the station; did you show empathy, did you listen actively and acknowledge? The use of both open and closed questions is important. Be sure to explore the 2nd ICE – Ideas, Concerns and Expectations – 'Any thoughts on what this could be?' 'Are you concerned about anything in particular?'

Summarise and then ensure that you have met the patient's expectations. 'This is the plan. Are you happy with what we have discussed/was this what you were expecting?'

Management plan: know your different types of discharges and the 1st line management for those.

Type of Discharge	What it may mean	Management
Bloody or brown	Irregular menstrual cycle, cancer?	Referral
Cloudy or yellow	Gonorrhoea	IM Ceftriaxone
Frothy, yellow or greenish with a bad odour	Trichomoniasis	Oral metronidazole
Pink	Lochia (shredding of the uterine lining after childbirth)	Conservative
Thick, white cottage cheese like	Yeast infection	Intravaginal cream/pessary – clotrimazole or oral fluconazole
White, grey, or yellow with fishy odour	Bacterial vaginosis	Oral metronidazole

FOCUSED DIAGNOSTIC HISTORY

Case Scenario 4

A 52-year-old man is your next patient in A&E. His wife found him on the bathroom floor with blood around his mouth. Take only a focused history and discuss the initial management plan with your senior. (NOTE: FOCUSED)

1 ICE – Introduction, Consent and Exposure (not needed in this scenario)

Introduce yourself: full name and your role

Confirm patient identity (name and date of birth)

Ask for consent: 'Is it okay if I take a history from you?' 'I understand you had a funny turn earlier, can you please tell me more about it?'

2 History of Presenting Complaint

Explore the cause of why the patient was lying on the floor and then why he had blood around his mouth

Most likely caused by vomiting blood (haematemesis)

Vomiting – ask how many episodes, how long for, quantity and the colour of the blood, has it happened before?

Any obvious cause of the vomiting?

Have you tried anything that has helped?

Explore upper gastrointestinal (GI) bleed causes:

Associated symptoms: recent change in bowel habits, abdominal pain, vomiting, relation to food, change in appetite, weight loss, dysphagia, bleeding from back passage- melaena

Red flags and systemic symptoms: weight loss, night sweats, fevers and pain elsewhere

Quick review of a general system review (if appropriate)

3 Past Medical History

Explore their past medical history so you can ask, 'Do you have any diagnosed medical conditions, such as peptic ulcers or reflux? Has this ever happened before? If so, how was it treated?' It is also good to ask about any past surgical history and about any bleeding disorders.

4 Drug History

It is ideal to ask about the drug history after asking about the past medical history. Always ask about anticoagulation/ anti-platelets if bleeding is involved. If the patient tells you they have been taking anti-inflammatories i.e. Ibuprofen or Naproxen long-term (ALARM BELLS), think suspected ruptured peptic ulcer causing the upper GI bleed? (NB ask about dosage, route, how many times a day)

Explore any allergies at this point.

5 Family History

Explore any family history here: 'Can I ask about any medical illnesses that run in your family?' – particularly any bleeding disorders.

6 Social History

Explore: smoking – pack years, alcohol intake, use of any recreational drugs, lifestyle, diet. Any physical fitness, occupation, any issues at home/stress related (if relevant)? (NB smoking, alcohol, poor diet, stress are all risk factors for peptic ulcers)

7 Travel history

Ask specifically about any recent travel abroad.

Additional Marks

This will depend on how you communicate the station: did you show empathy, did you listen actively and acknowledge. The use of both open and closed questions is important. Be sure to explore the 2nd ICE – Ideas, Concerns and Expectations – 'Any thoughts on what this could be?' 'Are you concerned about anything in particular?'

Summarise and then ensure that you have met the patient's expectations. 'This is the plan. Are you happy with what we have discussed/was this what you were expecting?'

Management plan: think about all your potential differentials for causes of vomiting blood (haematemesis)

- Mallory Weiss tears
- Oesophageal varices – cirrhosis, portal hypertension

- Aspirin overdose
- Ruptured peptic ulcer – causing upper GI bleed

Initial management will depend on severity if patient is haemodynamically unstable – a full A-approach should be used and possible fluid resuscitation/blood transfusion. Otherwise, patient should be admitted, BOXES:

B   Bloods (FBC, U&Es etc.)
O   Orifice testing- Sputum, urine, stool test for H. pylori (NB most common cause of peptic ulcers)
X   X-ray (chest x-ray)
E   ECG
S   Special test i.e. endoscopy

Be sure to suggest the use of scoring system: Rockall score.

1st line is to perform urgent endoscopy in unstable patients with severe acute upper GI bleeding.

Finally, if they mentioned they are on any long-term naproxen for arthritis, mention you would stop that medication.

SAFETY NET!

INFORMATION GIVING

Procedures

1 ICE – Introduction, Consent and Exposure (if needed)

Introduce yourself: full name and your role

Confirm patient identity (name and date of birth)

Confirm the reason for attendance, check their existing knowledge they have about the procedures and if they have followed the specific instructions prior to the procedure.

Before you start to explain, give them a quick structure about what you will talk about and tell them to feel free to ask any questions or to stop you at any time if they don't understand something.
For all procedures, when explaining:

- What is the procedure and what it will entail
- Reason for the procedure
- Process of procedure:
  – Before
  – During
  – After
- Risks + benefits of the procedure

Good procedures to go over are:

- Bronchoscopy
- Gastroscopy
- Colonoscopy
- Flexible sigmoidoscopy
- Cystoscopy
- Peak expiratory flow

Peak Expiratory Flow
(Remember – for all examination type stations
1 mark for washing/gelling hands)

1 ICE – Introduction, Consent and Exposure (not needed in this scenario)

Introduce yourself: full name and your role

Confirm patient identity (name and date of birth)

Check why they are here and gain consent to continue

2 Questions to ask before starting:

Check if patient has had a recent chest infection

When was the last time they used their inhalers or had a course of steroids?

3 Explain Procedure

It is a quick and easy test to see how well your lungs are working. You can explain and demonstrate at the same time:

- Stand up straight
- Take peak flow, bring dial to zero and hold it horizontally, do not cover the ends and do not block the dials
- Breath in and out to begin with
- Take a deep breath in
- Form a tight seal around the mouthpiece
- Blow out a quick sharp breath as hard as you can for about 10 seconds
- This should be repeated at least 3 times (however, if it aggravates asthma, once is sufficient), ensure to reset dial each time
- Inform patient that the best of 3 measurements will be used as the result

4 To Plot on Nomogram or Take Required Information for it

- Patient's height, weight, age and gender
- State that you will plot that on the gram and add to patient's notes
- To end you can ask patient to keep a record at home by taking their peak flow measurements once in the day and once in the night

5 Upon Completion of the Procedure

Wash hands, ask if they have any questions and thank the patient

Explaining a Diagnosis

To explain a diagnosis, you must understand the condition well. Note in the nationals they can ask about any condition. Most common ones are: hypertension, diabetes, benign prostatic hyperplasia, irritable bowel syndrome, inflammatory bowel disease, hypo/hyperthyroidism etc

1 ICE – Introduction, Consent and Exposure (if needed)

Introduce yourself: full name and your role

Confirm patient identity (name and date of birth)

Gain consent

Confirm the reason for attendance, check their existing knowledge. Explain what you will be talking about and let them know they can ask questions or ask you to repeat something if they don't understand.

2 Explain the normal

3 Explain the disease

4 Explain how it will affect the patient – symptoms, signs, any long-term complications

5 Explain the management

6 Check their understanding and ask if they have any questions or want you to repeat anything

7 Always provide a leaflet about condition and say 'I know I have given you a lot of information today, so here is a leaflet on what we spoke about'

8 If there is time, summarise and check understanding

9 Thank you

Explanation of a Medication

1 ICE – Introduction, Consent and Exposure (if needed)

Introduce yourself: full name and your role

Confirm patient identity (name and date of birth)

Gain consent

Confirm the reason for attendance, check their existing knowledge. Explain what you will be talking about and let them know they can ask questions or ask you to repeat something if they don't understand.

Always check contraindications of a medication i.e. is this patient pregnant?

Use ATHLETICS to remember to provide all relevant information about the drug, again remember any medication could be asked

A Action
T Timing
H How it works
L Length of treatment
E Effects – when it starts taking effect, when they may start to notice its effects
T Tests- monitoring i.e. for methotrexate
I Important side effects
C Complications
S Summary

MOTIVATIONAL INTERVIEWING

Smoking Cessation

1 ICE – Introduction, Consent and Exposure (not needed in this scenario)

Introduce yourself: full name and your role

Confirm patient identity (name and date of birth)

Confirm the reason for attendance, check their existing knowledge and their understanding of smoking and its associated health risks.

2 ICE – Ideas, Concerns and Expectations

You can ask these questions:

- 'How do you feel about smoking?'
- 'Is there anything that worries you about smoking or are you thinking of giving up?'
- 'What are you hoping to get from this visit today?'

Ensure to emphasise that this consultation is just a discussion and they can guide it through. Explain what you will be talking about and let them know they can ask questions or ask you to repeat something if they don't understand.

3 Smoking History

(If this information has already been given to you, please do not take a history. However, if not, then before a smoking cessation consultation a history is important.)

- How many years have they been smoking?
- How much does the patient smoke? (pack-years = [number of years smoked] x [average number of packs smoked per day]; one pack is equal to 20 cigarettes)
- What type of tobacco/nicotine do they use?
- How does smoking make them feel?
- Does smoking affect their life and interpersonal relationships?
- Have they previously tried to quit? If so, what resulted in the patient relapsing?
- Does the patient experience any withdrawal symptoms? (e.g. craving, irritability, dizziness, low mood, fatigue, insomnia)

4 Past Medical History and Drug History

Particularly smoking-related ones:

- Pre-existing lung disease (e.g. chronic obstructive pulmonary disease, asthma, pulmonary fibrosis)
- Cardiovascular disease and cardiovascular risk factors (e.g. coronary artery disease, hypertension, diabetes, hyperlipidaemia, stroke/TIA)
- Previous hospitalisation and surgery

Ask patient if they are currently or were previously prescribed any nicotine replacement therapy (NRT) and if so, how did they find it.

5 Family History

Ask about any illnesses that may run in the family

6 Social History

- Alcohol intake
- Any use of recreational drugs
- Psychosocial aspects of the patient's health including stressors at home, work, finances and support at home

7 The 5 As Approach:

ASK, ADVISE, ASSESS, ASSIST, ARRANGE:

- **Ask** – Identify smoking status for every patient at every visit, as this can always change
- **Advise** – Urge every smoker to try and quit. Praise the patient for coming in to discuss this. Advise the patient about the risks and complications of smoking, including the long-term effects i.e. cardiovascular disease, lung cancer etc.
- **Assess** – Is the patient wanting to quit and want more information on it? How much do they already know about the consequences of smoking? How motivated are they to quit? Use the 'Stages of Change' model for assessment *
- **Assist** – If the patient is willing to quit. Use the 'Star Approach'**
- **Arrange** – Arrange follow-up contact, in person or by telephone (preferably within the first week)

* **Stages of Change**

- Pre-contemplation: no interest in changing behaviour
- Contemplation: an awareness of the negative aspects of smoking
- Preparation: an understanding of why they should quit smoking
- Action maintenance: an attempt to stop smoking
- Relapse: the attempt to quit was unsuccessful

** **STAR Approach**

- **Set** a quit date
- **Tell** family and friends: patient to make family and friends aware that they are quitting, so they can get support and encouragement
- **Anticipate** challenges that they may face and make plans on how to overcome them.
- **Remove** all tobacco products such as ashtrays, lighters etc, also recommend counselling programmes and pharmacological therapies

Pharmacological Therapies

Nicotine replacement therapy (NRT):

- Used as first-line therapy and available in a variety of forms (e.g. patches, spray)
- Increases successful cessation by 1.5 times
- Caution in patients with cardiovascular disease or acute coronary syndrome

Bupropion:

- Increases successful cessation by 2 times
- Advise the patient to commence the medication for 1-2 weeks before the quit date and complete a 12-week course
- Contraindications: hypersensitivity reactions, seizure disorders and eating disorders

Varenicline:

- Works as a nicotine receptor partial agonist
- It is the most effective pharmacological therapy, increasing successful cessation by greater than 2 times
- Advise the patient to commence the medication 1 week before their quit date and complete a total course of 12 weeks
- Contraindications: hypersensitivity reactions

BREAKING BAD NEWS

Case Scenario

A 40-year-old female has been sent a letter by her GP to come and discuss her smear test results. Explain the results to her and the next steps.

The results show 'Positive for high-risk HPV and moderate dyskaryosis'

1 ICE – Introduction, Consent and Exposure (not needed in this scenario)

Introduce yourself: full name and your role

Confirm patient identity (name and date of birth)

Consent

Remember: SPIKES

2 S – Setting

Turn to the examiner and inform them that you would ensure the patient is comfortable and will ensure that the consultation takes place in an appropriate environment such as a side room. Also tell the examiner that you will remove all distraction from person, i.e. bleep/phone in an hospital setting and in GP will ensure to have an extended appointment with the patient and to let staff know not to disturb.

Offer to have someone else with them in the room for support, ask the patient if they want a family member or friend to be there with them.

3 P – Perspective

Check with the patient what they already know and what they are expecting from today's consultation. At that point ask what has led them to this consultation, i.e. any symptoms or what has been going on so far.

Ensure to pick up on any verbal or non-verbal cues from the patient, try gauge the patient's current emotional state.

4 I – Invitation

Always check if the patient wants to receive their results today and will they like full details or would prefer to receive them when with a family or friend for support. 'Is it okay for me to tell you/talk about the results today?'

At this point you can explain a plan of how this consultation will go: 'So, I will talk about your results, what they mean and what we will need to do next.'

5 K – Knowledge

Key is to always open up with a warning, that you are about to disclose some 'bad news', before actually breaking the news.

Slowly disclose the news, but in sizeable chunks to allow the patient to take in what you are telling them. Keep checking their understanding so far and remember to let the patient's emotions be a guide. DO NOT deliver the news like a robot. Deal with what you have in front of you. Ensure to allow for reasonable pauses.

Avoid the use of jargon. If required, always explain or describe what it means or entails.

6 E – Empathy and Emotion

Disclose the news in a respectful manner and ensure to have a clear and slow pace in your tone.

Empathy is key, which can pass or fail your station. Deal with what is in front of you. Acknowledge and verbalise the stress of the situation that they may be feeling.

7 S – Strategy and Summary

Summarise everything you have discussed and check the patient has understood.

Make a plan together and discuss what the next step will be.

Reassure them that the necessary referral and steps will be taken accordingly and explain that you may not have all the answers now. You can say 'I know you may have a lot of questions but I don't want to give you information that is out of my remit. I can understand this may be frustrating but you can write your questions down and take them with you when you see the specialist.'

End with checking the patient's understanding and direct them towards possible leaflets on e.g investigation etc.

Offer to help break news to family and friends and check support network. Direct them to support groups if appropriate.

8 TIPS

- Ensure to be respectful and empathetic throughout
- Have a slow and clear tone
- Size and chunk – deliver information is small chunks, allowing for pauses in between
- Explore ideas, concerns and expectations
- Active listening is key and provide appropriate eye contact
- Professional body language (leaning slightly forward in the chair, arms and legs uncrossed)
- Nodding and acknowledging
- Do not interrupt the patient and build rapport by checking on how they are feeling

DEALING WITH CONFLICT

Case Scenario

A patient has been awaiting physiotherapy referral and he was just told by the receptionist that the previous clinician had not processed the referral. The patient is very angry and has been booked in to see you this afternoon.

BEFORE YOU BEGIN: state to the examiner that you will check that you are safe and close to the door, aware of alarm button, etc.

1 ICE – Introduction, Consent and Exposure (not needed in this scenario)

Introduce yourself: full name and your role

Confirm patient identity (name and date of birth)

Consent for consultation (Note patient's current body language and expressions)

2 Confirm

Confirm what they have come in for:

'Can I ask you to confirm why you have come to see us today, please?'

3 Listen

This is very important. Let the patient say everything they want and do not interrupt or patronise them. They may get very upset when doing this. Remember to stay calm and let the patient vent.

4 Recognise

Recognise that they are getting upset and angry, make an acknowledgement: 'I can see this is making you quite upset.' 'I am sorry that the referral to physiotherapy hasn't been made, I will try and look into this for you.'

5 More Information

Ask any further details if required. Don't make assumptions on why the patient is angry, always let them explain why and direct the dialogue accordingly.

6 Apologise

Ensure that you apologise for the situation but DO NOT take the blame: 'I am sorry this has happened.'

Reassure them and tell them you will try to look into it and investigate what has happened.

DO NOT agree or guarantee that you will fix this: 'I will look into this for you and try get it sorted'. If you are able to do it during the consultation then do so. However, if there are time constraints, then come up with an agreement with patient, 'I will contact you once I know more.' If it's a different scenario where it is regarding diagnosis etc, do not give out information you are not sure about.

7 Check

Check they are happy with the plan and ask if they have any more questions.

TELEPHONE COMMUNICATION – HAND OVER

SBAR – Situation, Background, Assessment, Recommend/Refer

Case Scenario 1

Mrs Ghopal is a 52-year-old woman who was diagnosed with heart failure 4 years ago. She has come into hospital today at 2.25pm with shortness of breath (SOB). She says that she ran out of her medications 2 days ago. On examination, she is alert and orientated. When you ask her to stand up, she is short of breath (SOB on exertion), oxygen saturation is 88% on room air. On auscultation you hear fine bibasal crackles. When examining her limbs, you note some lower limb peripheral oedema bilaterally. Observations: T- 37.2, BP- 135/88, PR- 125, RR- 34/min.

You are asked to arrange for cardiology review for this patient. Please call the on-call cardiologist and arrange for this.

When outside, mark and highlight the SBAR. You will be able to take the paper in with you. If you have marked SBAR then you will be able to hand over in the correct format.

1 Situation

- Introduce yourself: name, role and department you are working in
- Ask who you are speaking to
- Identify the patient you want to discuss or handover (their name, dob/age, hospital ID and gender)
- Your reason for the call – what you need advice on or what you need

2 Background

- Using the scenario, take the pertinent past medical history, so here: 'today at 2.25pm'
- The reason of attendance, the presenting complaint and current issues and current treatment, if any

3 Assessment

- What you have done so far i.e. the treatment
- The current ABCDE, the observations and if any investigations have been done – their results if at hand, otherwise state just the investigations that have been carried out

4 Recommend/refer

- Ask what you want; here, 'I would like you to come and see this patient as he requires a cardiology review'
- If you don't know what the problem is then be honest

2

Examination Skills

YOU WONT BE EXPECTED TO TALK THROUGH THE ENTIRE STATION, BUT YOU CAN MENTION KEY POINTS AND ENSURE TO ALWAYS ALLOW FOR SOME TIME AT THE END TO SUMMARISE YOUR POSITIVE AND NEGATIVE FINDINGS.

VITAL SIGNS / EARLY WARNING SCORE

Case Scenario 1

This 32-year-old man has been admitted and moved to the Acute medical unit. Please take all the necessary vital signs and record them accordingly.

1 ICE – Introduction, Consent and Exposure

Introduce yourself: full name and your role

Confirm patient identity (name and date of birth)

Explain the examination

Consent for examination

Appropriate position and exposure

Always ask about chaperone

Wash/gel hands

2 General Inspection

Patient: state if they look well, their colour, pallor/flushing, any shortness of breath/audible wheeze

Surroundings: oxygen mask, IV lines, medication

3 Examination

Ensure to inform your patient at every step what you are doing or are about to do

Respiratory Rate: calculate the respiratory rate (counting rise and fall of chest), pretend to take the pulse, so patient doesn't become conscious of their own breathing. Measure for at least 15-30 seconds and then times by 4 to get to 60 seconds.

Heart Rate: measure heart rate at radial pulse. Measure for at least 15-30 seconds and then times by 4 to get to 60 seconds.

Oxygen Saturations: measure using pulse oximeter provided (check heart rate against reading on pulse oximeter if necessary)

Temperature: measure temperature using provided probe

Blood Pressure: Select appropriate cuff size if there are different sizes

Position cuff at appropriate level (2cm above antecubital fossa)

Centre bladder over the brachial artery and wrap cuff tight (do not cause discomfort)

Inflate cuff, palpating artery to detect at which pressure the pulse disappears

Deflate cuff and wait 30 seconds

Relocate brachial artery and position stethoscope over it

Inflate cuff to 30 mm Hg above palpated systolic pressure

Slowly release valves

Accurately identify pulse within 10mm Hg both systolic and diastolic

AVPU: note patient's level of alertness (alert, voice, pain, unresponsive)

4 To Complete

Offer to perform lying/standing blood pressure (if appropriate)

Complete the NEWS chart to an adequate sufficiency (do not forget to total NEWS score)

Summarise findings in logical and structured manner

Offer diagnosis and differential diagnoses if appropriate

CALCULATING A BMI

Make sure all the measurements are in the correct format to calculate the body mass index (BMI)

This is the formula: $BMI = kg/m^2$

Example: The patient's weight is 68kg and their height is 165cm, what is their BMI?

Remember to convert cm into m
165cm = 1.65m
$BMI = 68 / 1.65^2 = 24.98$

LUMPS AND BUMPS

1 ICE – Introduction, Consent and Exposure

Introduce yourself: full name and your role

Confirm patient identity (name and date of birth)

Explain the examination: 'Today I will need to examine the lump on your...'

Explain that it shouldn't be painful, but may be uncomfortable. If they want you to stop at any point, to let you know and you will stop.

Consent for examination

Appropriate position and exposure

Always ask about chaperone. If it's an intimate examination, always have a chaperone present.

Wash/gel hands

Always check for pain before starting

2 General Inspection

Patient: state if they look well, their colour, pallor/flushing, any shortness of breath/do they look like they are in pain

Surroundings: oxygen mask, IV lines, medication, vomit bowls

3 Close Inspection, Palpation, Auscultation if necessary

Remember: SPACEPIT

S   SIZE
P   POSITION (site)
A   ATTACHMENT
C   CONSISTENCY/CONTOUR
E   EDGES
P   PULSATION
I   INFLAMMATION
T   TRANSLUMINANCE

SIZE: use a tape measure if available (otherwise, a shortcut is to measure and memorise the length of the distal phalanx of your index finger, and use that as a reference).

POSITION: be precise, if there are multiple lumps, this is more suggestive of superficial lymph nodes, superficial lesions (e.g. lipoma) or dermatological problems (e.g. large skin lesions).

ATTACHMENT: is the lump freely mobile, or is it tethered to a structure such as skin or muscle? Malignant lumps are often fixed to surrounding tissue.

CONSISTENCY: comment whether the lump is hard, firm, soft or nodular. Hard corresponds to the feel of your forehead, firm to the tip of your nose, and soft to your lip.

CONTOUR: this refers to the look and texture of the skin overlying the lump. Is it the same as the rest of the skin, or thick/rough/scaly/smooth/shiny?

EDGES: this refers to the whole outline of the lump (e.g. round/oval/irregular/well-defined)

PULSATION: is the lump pulsatile? Pulsatility suggests underlying vascular aetiology (e.g. an aneurysm).

INFLAMMATION: palpate the temperature using the back of your hand, comparing to surrounding tissue. Significantly increased temperature suggests infection (e.g. abscess) and will normally be associated with erythema. Is the lump a different colour from the surrounding skin (e.g. erythematous)?

TRANSLUMINANCE: ideally dim the lights in the room first. Shine a light through the lump and see if it illuminates. Transillumination suggests that the lump is cystic (e.g. hydrocoele).

Other tests

Compressibility

- This test should only be used for suspected hernias
- Check if the lump can be compressed (reduced)
- You can ask the patient to do this, or do it yourself
- If the lump can be reduced completely, it may only reappear if the patient increases pressure (e.g. by coughing)
- You can ask the patient to lie down and if the lump reduces spontaneously, this makes the diagnosis of a hernia highly likely
- Hernias are typically reducible; however, if a hernia is painful and irreducible it suggests that it is strangulated (this is a surgical emergency)

Cough impulse

- This test should be used for suspected hernias
- Ask the patient to cough whilst you palpate the lump
- A positive cough impulse occurs when you see and/or feel the lump increase in size when the patient coughs
- A cough impulse indicates a communication between the intra-abdominal cavity and the lump (e.g. a hernia)

To complete the examination

- Thank the patient
- Allow the patient time to get dressed
- Suggest a differential diagnosis for the lump (common lumps in OSCEs include hernias, lipomas, neck lumps)

Summarise findings:

Example

> 'Mrs A has a single lump in the anterior wall of her right axilla. It is a defined sphere around 4cm across. It is very red, hot and tender on palpation. The lump is non-pulsatile with no bruit. My findings are consistent with a suspected abscess.'

Thank patient and wash hands.

FOR all musculoskeletal (MSK) examinations remember: LOOK, FEEL, MOVE and SPECIAL TESTS

HAND EXAMINATION

1 ICE – Introduction, Consent and Exposure

Introduce yourself: full name and your role

Confirm patient identity (name and date of birth)

Consent for examination: 'Is it okay for me to examine your hand/wrists today?'

Explain the examination

Appropriate position and exposure (to expose both arms above the elbows). If there is a pillow available, use it to rest patient's arms.

Always ask about chaperone

Wash/gel hands

Always check for pain before starting, acknowledge pain and say, 'I can see you are in pain, hopefully we can get you sorted soon.' Ask if they would like any pain relief and say you will arrange for some after the examination.

2 General Inspection

Patient: state if they look well, their colour, pallor/flushing, do they look like they are in pain, obvious trauma

Surroundings: oxygen mask, IV lines, medication, mobility aids, splint/cast

3 Look

State at least 3 things you would look for in each part/area

Dorsal: scars, erythema/pallor, swelling, Bouchard's nodes, Heberden's nodes, boutonnieres deformity, swan neck deformity, Z-thumb deformity, bruising, muscle wasting, nail pitting,

Palmar: asymmetry, erythema/pallor, thenar/hypothenar wasting, Dupuytren's contracture

Extensor surface of arm: psoriatic plaques, rheumatoid nodules

4 Feel/palpate

State at least 3 things you would palpate for in each part/area

Check for pain before starting

Dorsal: temperature, palpate individual joints (swelling, effusions, synovitis, deformities), palpate anatomical snuffbox, perform MCP squeeze, palpate for tendon tenderness

Palmar: palpate thenar/hypothenar bulk, palpate for tendon thickening

Wrist: palpate for joint line irregularities, tenderness

5 Move

Do all movements – ensure to do passive and active movements

Wrist: flexion and extension (pain/crepitus felt when moving), pronation, supination, radial and ulnar deviation

Fingers: active and passive flexion and extension (pain/crepitus) in all fingers

Thumb: extension, resisted abduction, opposition, adduction

Function: power grip, pincer grip

6 Special Tests

Offer to perform Phalen's test (reverse prayer sign for 1 min)

Offer to perform Tinel's test (tap median nerve in wrist)

Offer to telescope the thumb (particularly in suspecting scaphoid fracture) – hold thumb firmly and push it into the wrist)

7 To Complete

Summarise findings in logical and structured manner

Offer appropriate diagnosis and differential diagnoses

Further investigations: elbow examination, upper neurological examination, x-ray i.e. scaphoid views 4 in total if suspecting scaphoid fracture or presenting with fall on outstretched hand (FOOSH)

Offer a leaflet on possible hand/wrist injuries

Thank the patient

Wash hands

8 Tips

- When discussing possible diagnosis and management, the common ones for OSCEs are carpal tunnels, scaphoid fractures (Note it could be any pathology)
- Know the 1st line management at least, i.e. for scaphoid fracture – splinting for at least 6 weeks and that not all fractures show up on x-ray, therefore repeat in 2 weeks if still symptomatic, possible MRI?

SPINE EXAMINATION

1 ICE – Introduction, Consent and Exposure

Introduce yourself: full name and your role

Confirm patient identity (name and date of birth)

Consent for examination: 'Is it okay for me to examine your spine and back today?'

Explain the examination

Appropriate position and exposure (to expose back, remove top, from waist upwards)

Always ask about chaperone

Wash/gel hands

Always check for pain before starting, acknowledge pain and say, 'I can see you are in pain, hopefully we can get you sorted.' Ask if they would like any pain relief and say you will arrange for some after the examination.

2 General Inspection

Patient: state if they look well, their colour, pallor/flushing, do they look like they are in pain, obvious trauma, any obvious deformities, scoliosis, lordosis, scars, muscle wasting, asymmetry

Surroundings: mobility aids, splint/cast/plasters

3 Look

Ask the patient to **stand** and **turn in 90° increments** as you inspect the spine from each angle

Anterior inspection

- Scars
- **Posture:** note any asymmetry which may indicate joint pathology or scoliosis
- **Asymmetry of the shoulder girdle:** may be caused by scoliosis, arthritis, fractures or dislocation
- **Pelvic tilt:** lateral pelvic tilt can be caused by scoliosis
- Lateral inspection
- **Cervical lordosis:** hyper lordosis is associated osteoarthritis
- **Thoracic kyphosis:** hyper kyphosis is associated with Scheuermann's disease (congenital wedging of the vertebrae)
- **Lumbar lordosis:** loss of normal lumbar lordosis is associated with sacroiliac joint disease (e.g. ankylosing spondylitis)

Posterior inspection

- **Spinal alignment:** inspect for lateral curvature of the spine indicative of scoliosis.
- **Iliac crest alignment:** misalignment may indicate a leg length discrepancy or hip abductor weakness
- **Muscle wasting:** note any wasting of the paraspinal muscles which may indicate chronic spinal pathology and reduced mobility
- **Abnormal hair growth:** may indicate underlying bony abnormalities such as spina bifida

4 Feel/palpate

Check for pain before starting

Check gait: ask them to walk – describe i.e. antalgic

Palpate spinous processes of all vertebra (start from the c-spine) and sacroiliac joints, assessing their alignment and noting any tenderness.

Palpate paraspinal muscles for tenderness (start from the top) do one side at a time and support the other while doing so.

5 Move

Do all movements – ensure to do passive and active movements

Cervical

Flexion

Instructions: ask the patient to touch their chin to their chest

Extension

Instructions: ask the patient to look up at the ceiling.

Lateral

Instructions: ask the patient to touch their ear to their shoulder on each side

Rotation

Instructions: ask the patient to turn their head to the left and the right.

Lumbar spine

Flexion

Instructions: ask the patient to touch their toes whilst keeping their legs straight.

Extension

Instructions: ask the patient to lean back as far as they are comfortably able, whilst you're positioned close to them for support if required.

Lateral flexion

Instructions: ask the patient to slide their left hand down the outer aspect of their left leg as far as they are able to whilst keeping their legs straight. Then ask them to repeat by sliding their right hand over their right leg.

Thoracic spine

Instructions: ask the patient to sit on the side of the clinical examination couch and cross their arms across their chest. Then ask them to turn to the left and the right as far as they are comfortably able to.

6 Special Tests

Schober's test

Schober's test can be used to identify **restricted flexion of the lumbar spine**

- Identify the location of the posterior superior iliac spine (PSIS) on each side.
- Mark the skin in the midline 5cm below the PSIS.
- Mark the skin in the midline 10cm above the PSIS.
- Ask the patient to touch their toes to assess lumbar flexion.
- Measure the distance between the two lines.

If a patient has **normal lumbar flexion** the **distance** between the **two marks** should **increase** from the initial 15cm to **more than 20cm**

Reduced range of motion is associated with conditions such as **ankylosing spondylitis**.

Sciatic stretch test (a.k.a. straight leg raise)

The **sciatic stretch test** is used to identify **sciatic nerve irritation**

- Position the patient supine on the clinical examination couch.
- Holding the patient's ankle, raise their leg by passively flexing the hip whilst keeping the patient's knee fully extended.
- The normal range of movement for passive hip flexion is approximately 80-90°.
- Once the patient's hip is flexed, dorsiflex the patient's foot.

The **sciatic stretch test** is considered **positive** if the patient experiences **pain in the posterior thigh** or **buttock region**.

A positive test is suggestive of **sciatic nerve irritation** (e.g. secondary to lumbar disc prolapse).

7 To Complete

Summarise findings in logical and structured manner

Offer appropriate diagnosis and differential diagnoses

Further investigations: to examine the shoulder and hip, imaging

Offer a leaflet on possible spinal/back problems

Thank the patient

Wash hands

TIPS

- To end always say you will assess the joint above and below to complete the examination

HIP EXAMINATION

1 ICE – Introduction, Consent and Exposure

Introduce yourself: full name and your role

Confirm patient identity (name and date of birth)

Consent for examination: 'Is it okay for me to examine your hips today?'

Explain the examination

Appropriate position and exposure (to expose to underwear)

Always ask about chaperone

Wash/gel hands

Always check for pain before starting, acknowledge pain and say, 'I can see you are in pain, hopefully we can get you sorted soon.' Ask if they would like any pain relief and say you will arrange for some after the examination.

2 General Inspection

Patient: state if they look well, their colour, pallor/flushing, do they look like they are in pain, obvious trauma, any obvious deformities, asymmetry

Surroundings: mobility aids, splint/cast/plasters, wheelchair

Gait: speed, stride length, antalgic/Trendelenburg gait? Footwear

3 Look

Front: temperature, scars, pelvic tilt, quadriceps wasting, foot deformity

Side: temperature, stoop, lumbar lordosis, scars, temperature

Behind: temperature, gluteal atrophy

4 Feel

Palpate greater trochanter, anterior superior iliac spine, around joint (tenderness/temperature/effusion)

Measure real leg length (anterior superior iliac spine to medial malleolus)

Measure apparent leg length (xiphisternum to medial malleolus)

5 Move

Active and passive flexion, passive extension (on the front, assess range)

Passive internal and external rotation

Passive abduction and adduction

6 Special Tests

Offer to perform Thomas's test

Thomas's test: to assess for a **fixed flexion deformity** (i.e. an inability for the patient to fully extend their leg).

- With the patient positioned flat on the bed, place a hand below their lumbar spine with your palm facing upwards (this helps to prevent the patient from masking a fixed flexion deformity by increasing lumbar lordosis).
- Passively flex the hip of the unaffected leg as far as you are able to and observe the contralateral limb.
- Repeat the assessment on the contralateral hip.

Interpretation

The test is **positive** (abnormal) if the **affected thigh raises off the bed**, indicating a **loss of hip joint extension**. This would suggest a **fixed flexion deformity** in the affected hip.

Offer to illicit Trendelenburg's sign

Trendelenburg's test

Trendelenburg's test is used to screen for **hip abductor weakness**

- With the patient upright, stand in front of them and ask them to place their hands on your forearms or shoulders for stability.
- Position your fingers on each side of the patient's pelvis at the iliac crest.
- Ask the patient to stand on one leg and observe your fingers for evidence of lateral pelvic tilt.
- Repeat the assessment with the patient standing on the other leg.

Interpretation

If the patient's hip abductors are functioning **normally** the pelvis should **remain stable** or **rise slightly on the side of the raised leg**.

If the **pelvis drops on the side of the raised leg** it suggests **contralateral hip abductor weakness** (this is known as Trendelenburg's sign).

7 To Complete

Summarise findings in logical and structured manner

Offer appropriate diagnosis and differential diagnoses

Further investigations: to examine the spine and knees, imaging and lower limb neurological examination

Offer a leaflet on possible hip problems i.e. osteoarthritis (know 1st line management i.e. paracetamol)

Thank the patient

Wash hands

KNEE EXAMINATION

1 ICE – Introduction, Consent and Exposure

Introduce yourself: full name and your role

Confirm patient identity (name and date of birth)

Consent for examination: 'Is it okay for me to examine your knees today?'

Explain the examination

Appropriate position and exposure (to expose to underwear)

Always ask about chaperone

Wash/gel hands

Always check for pain before starting, acknowledge pain and say, 'I can see you are in pain, hopefully we can get you sorted.' Ask if they would like any pain relief and say you will arrange for some after the examination.

2 General Inspection

Patient: state if they look well, their colour, pallor/flushing, do they look like they are in pain, obvious trauma, any obvious deformities, asymmetry

Surroundings: mobility aids, splint/cast/plasters, wheelchair

Gait: speed, antalgic gait? Footwear

3 Look

Look from front, side and back

Front: swelling, red, deformity

Side: asymmetry

Back: swelling (popliteal/baker's cyst)

4 Feel

Check temperature, muscle bulk around joint,

Palpate medial and lateral joint line with knees flexed

Palpate borders of patellar and checks for patellar effusion

5 Move

Assess active and passive flexion

Assess active and passive extension

Assess for pain/crepitus

6 Special Tests

Cruciate ligaments

Patient's knee flexed to 90 degrees

Correctly performs anterior and posterior draw test

State intention to perform McMurrays test for possible meniscal damage

Inform patient when examination is finished and if requiring any help putting their clothing back on

Collateral ligaments

Knee flexed to about 30 degrees

Correctly applies valgus stress with stabilisation of thigh proximal to knee and palpation of the medial knee

Correctly applies varus stress with stabilisation of thigh proximal to knee and palpation of the lateral knee

7 To Complete

Summarise findings in logical and structured manner

Offer appropriate diagnosis and differential diagnoses

Further investigations: to examine the hips and ankles, imaging and lower limb neurological examination

Offer a leaflet on possible knee problems

Thank the patient

Wash hands

SHOULDER EXAMINATION

1 ICE – Introduction, Consent and Exposure

Introduce yourself: full name and your role

Confirm patient identity (name and date of birth)

Consent for examination: 'Is it okay for me to examine your shoulders today?'

Explain the examination

Appropriate position and exposure (to expose shoulders)

Always ask about chaperone

Wash/gel hands

Always check for pain before starting, acknowledge pain and say, 'I can see you are in pain, hopefully we can get you sorted soon.' Ask if they would like any pain relief and say you will arrange for some after the examination.

2 General Inspection

Patient: state if they look well, their colour, pallor/flushing, do they look like they are in pain, obvious trauma, any obvious deformities, asymmetry

Surroundings: mobility aids, splint/cast/plasters/slings

3 Look

Anterior: asymmetry, scars, deltoid muscle wasting, swelling

Lateral: scars, swelling

Posterior: asymmetry, scars, para-vertebral/trapezius/deltoid muscle wasting, scoliosis, winged scapula

4 Feel

Assess joint temperature (both sides)

Palpate sternoclavicular joint, clavicle, AC joint, coracoid process, humeral head, greater tuberosity of humerus, spine of scapula (swelling tenderness)

5 Move

Active: flexion, extension, external rotation, internal rotation, abduction, adduction, assess movement of the scapula

Passive: flexion, extension, external rotation, internal rotation, abduction, adduction, internal and external rotation against resistance

6 Special Tests

Test for subacromial impingement – Hawkin's test (abduct arm to 90° and mimic emptying can)

Painful arc – (passive abduction to maximum point then actively lower arm)

Scarf ACJ test (place hand on opposite shoulder)

Rotator cuff tests

Supraspinatus – Jobe's test: (also known as 'empty can' test): arm abducted to 20 degrees, in the plane of the scapula, thumb pointing down

Infraspinatus and Teres minor: resisted external rotation with the arms by side

Subscapularis: Gerber's lift off test: push examiner's hand away from 'hand behind back position' (eliminates pectoralis major)

7 To Complete

Summarise findings in logical and structured manner

Offer appropriate diagnosis and differential diagnoses

Further investigations: to examine the spine and elbows, imaging and upper limb neurological examination

Offer a leaflet on possible shoulder problems, such as impingement, tears etc.

Thank the patient

Wash hands

HOW TO DESCRIBE A RASH

Always start with ICE

1 Size of the Lesion

Measure their width and height

2 Configuration of the Lesion

The shape or outline of skin lesions:

- **Discrete lesions:** individual lesions, clearly separated from one another (e.g. normal mole)
- **Confluent lesions:** lesions that appear to be merging together (e.g. urticaria)
- **Linear lesions:** lesions in the shape of a line (e.g. excoriations)
- **Discoid lesions:** coin-shaped lesions (e.g. discoid eczema, discoid lupus)
- **Target lesions:** concentric rings of varying colour, resembling a bullseye (e.g. erythema multiforme)
- **Annular lesions:** ring-like lesions (e.g. tinea corporis)

3 Colour of the Lesion

Colour examples

Erythematous lesions: redness of the skin caused by an increased blood supply to the area. Erythematous lesions will blanch when pressure is applied.

Purpuric lesions: reddish/purple discolouration of the skin caused by small blood vessels bleeding into the skin. Purpuric lesions do not blanch when pressure is applied. Petechiae are small purpuric lesions less than 2mm in diameter whereas ecchymoses are larger purpura more than 2mm across (commonly referred to as a bruise).

Hyperpigmented lesions: areas of darker skin caused by excess melanin production. Hyperpigmentation may be diffuse (e.g. Addison's disease) or discrete (linea nigra in pregnancy).

4 Morphology of the Lesion

Do the lesions appear flat, raised above the plane of the skin or depressed below it?

Primary lesions

Primary skin lesions are those which develop as a **direct result** of a **disease process**

Macule: a flat area of altered colour less than 1.5cm in diameter

Patch: a flat area of altered colour greater than 1.5cm in diameter

Papule: a solid raised palpable lesion less than 0.5cm in diameter

Nodule: a solid raised palpable lesion greater than 0.5cm in diameter

Plaque: a palpable flat lesion usually greater than 1cm in diameter

Vesicle: a raised, clear fluid-filled lesion less than 0.5cm in diameter

Bulla: a raised, clear fluid-filled lesion greater than 0.5cm in diameter

Pustule: a pus-containing lesion less than 0.5cm in diameter

Abscess: a localised accumulation of pus

Wheal: an oedematous papule or plaque caused by dermal oedema

Boil/furuncle: staphylococcal infection around or within a hair follicle

Carbuncle: staphylococcal infection of adjacent hair follicles (i.e. multiple boils/furuncles)

Secondary lesions

Secondary lesions are **modifications** of **primary lesions** that occur due to **trauma** to, or **evolution** of, the **primary lesion**.

Excoriation: loss of epidermis associated with trauma

Lichenification: thickening of the epidermis with exaggeration of normal skin lines, typically caused by chronic rubbing or scratching of an area (e.g. chronic eczema)

Scales: visible fragments of the stratum corneum as it is shed from the skin, most commonly associated with psoriasis

Crust: a rough surface consisting of dried serum, blood, bacteria and cellular debris. The serum, blood, bacteria and debris has usually exuded through an eroded epidermis.

Scar: new fibrous tissue which occurs after skin injury. Atrophic scarring involves the thinning of normal tissues underlying the scar resulting in a cratering effect.

Ulcer: a localised defect in the skin of irregular size and shape where the epidermis and some dermis have been lost. Ulcers ultimately result in scarring when healed.

Striae (stretch marks): purple lines on the skin caused by tearing during the rapid growth or overstretching of skin (e.g. growth spurts, ascites, intrabdominal malignancy, Cushing's syndrome, obesity, pregnancy). They undergo an evolution of colour from purple to pink to white as they mature.

5 Pigmented Lesion – ABCDE Approach

Asymmetry

Assess the **symmetry** of the **skin lesion**: asymmetry is suggestive of malignancy.

Border irregularity

Assess the **borders** of the **skin lesion**: note if they appear well-defined. Poorly defined borders are suggestive of malignancy.

Colour variation or changes

Assess the **colour** of the **skin lesion**: note if the colour appears consistent throughout the lesion. The presence of multiple colours within a single skin lesion is suggestive of malignancy.

Diameter

Assess the **diameter** of the **skin lesion**: measure the size of the skin lesion and ask the patient if it has been growing in size. Progressively enlarging skin lesions, particularly those over 6mm in diameter, are suggestive of malignancy.

Elevation/evolution

Assess the **elevation** of the **skin lesion** and **take a history** of the **lesion's evolution**: elevated skin lesions and those which have a history of bleeding and itching are more concerning for malignancy.

LYMPHORETICULAR EXAMINATION

1 ICE – Introduction, Consent and Exposure

Introduce yourself: full name and your role

Confirm patient identity (name and date of birth)

Consent for examination: 'Is it okay for me to examine some of the glands in your body today?'

Explain the examination

Appropriate position and exposure

Always ask about chaperone

Wash/gel hands

2 General Inspection

Patient: pallor, any obvious bruising or bleeding under skin, if patient looks unwell, any abdominal distension, obvious neck swelling

Surroundings: oxygen, IV drips, medication

3 Cervical Lymph Nodes

Stand behind the patient and use both hands to start palpating the neck, note any asymmetry in size, consistency and mobility of lymph nodes.

Start from submental area, submandibular, pre-auricular, post-auricular, anterior cervical, posterior cervical, occipital, supraclavicular

4 Axillary Lymph Nodes

Cover the pectoral (anterior), central (medial), subscapular (posterior), humoral (lateral), and apical groups of lymph nodes.

- Pectoral/anterior: with your palm facing towards you, palpate behind the lateral edge of the pectoralis major
- Central/medial: turn your palm medially and with your fingertips at the apex of the axilla palpate against the wall of the thorax
- Subscapular/posterior: facing your palm away from you now, feel inside the lateral edge of latissimus dorsi
- Humoral/lateral: palpate the inner aspect of the arm in the axilla
- Apex of the axilla with fingertips (warn the patient this may be uncomfortable).
- Repeat on the contralateral axilla.

5 Epitrochlear Lymph Nodes

Use your thumb to reach across the crease of the elbow to palpate the inner aspect of the arm just above the medial epicondyle of the humerus. (Ensure to examine both sides)

6 Inguinal Lymph Nodes (unlikely to do this in an OSCE, but mention it)

Palpate immediately inferior to the inguinal ligament (which runs between the anterior superior iliac spine and pubic tubercle)

7 Abdomen

Observe for:

- Scars, striae
- Masses
- Distension
- Pulsation
- Stomas
- Pulsations
- Palpate in all 9 regions (light and deep palpation), check for organomegaly

8 To Complete

Summarise findings in logical and structured manner

Offer appropriate diagnosis and differential diagnoses

Further investigations: BOXES

Offer a leaflet

Thank the patient

Wash hands

CARDIOVASCULAR EXAMINATION

1 ICE – Introduction, Consent and Exposure

Introduce yourself: full name and your role

Confirm patient identity (name and date of birth)

Consent for examination

Explain the examination: explain what you will be doing, so looking at hands, face, chest and legs, listening to the heart and checking pulses around the body

Appropriate position and exposure: 45° and expose chest (NB DO NOT use the word 'expose'). You can say, 'I will need you to remove all clothing (including your bra) from the waist upwards.'

Always ask about chaperone

Wash/gel hands

Always check for pain before starting, acknowledge pain and say, 'I can see you are in pain, hopefully we can get you sorted.' Ask if they would like any pain relief and say you will arrange for some after the examination.

2 General Inspection

Patient: in pain, pallor, malar flush, short of breath, obvious scars, pacemaker, peripheral oedema

Surroundings: oxygen masks, IV drips, ECG/heart monitors

3 Examination (NB Know all landmarks for pulses around the body)

Hands: clubbing – ask them to do Schamroth's window – signs for many conditions, signs for bacterial/infective endocarditis – Janeway lesions (painless red lesions in palm), Osler nodes (painful nodes on finger tips) and splinter haemorrhages in the nails, peripheral cyanosis, tendon xanthoma- hyperlipidaemia, and check for capillary refill – count out loud for 5 seconds and mention capillary refill return time. Check temperature of both hands.

Wrists: record the radial pulse (time for 15 seconds and then multiply number by 4). Comment on the rate, rhythm, volume. Check for radio-radial delay, and mention you can also check for radio- femoral delay – sign for aortic coarctation.

Arms: take both brachial pulses – comment on rate, rhythm and volume.

Check for collapsing pulse – aortic regurgitation (always check for pain in the shoulder and lift arm while fingers are on radial pulse). Positive sign is when the pulse weakens and comes back bounding.

Offer to check blood pressure

Neck: take the carotid pulse, one at a time, as bilateral palpation of carotid pulses simultaneously can compromise the arterial blood flow to the brain and stimulate the vagus nerve leading to vagal syncope. (Comment on rate, rhythm, volume.)

Check the jugular venous pressure (JVP). Positive sign will indicate right-sided heart failure. Ensure that the patient is lying back supine at 45° angle, observe the JVP and offer to measure (you would measure from the sternal angle, it should be less than 3-4cm). Offer to do the hepatojugular reflex to further extenuate the JVP (always check for abdominal pain before palpating).

Eyes: corneal arcus (can be normal finding in over 50s, otherwise consider hyperlipidaemia) xanthelasma – also a sign of hyperlipidaemia, conjunctival pallor – sign of anaemia.

Face: malar flush – sign of mitral stenosis

Mouth: ask patient to open mouth, check dental hygiene in relation to infective endocarditis, and ask them to raise their tongue to check for a high arched palate – sign of Marfan's syndrome. Check for central cyanosis and for angular stomatitis on the corners of the mouth – sign of iron deficiency.

Chest inspection: any obvious scars, visible apex beat, pacemaker, pacing wires

Chest palpation: palpate for the apex beat (NB to know anatomy for heart sounds) 5th intercostal space, midclavicular line. Heaves – use base of the hands over parasternal line (Present in right ventricular hypertrophy) an impulse like sensation that can lift hands. Thrills are palpable murmurs using base of fingers, feels like a vibration.

Chest auscultation: auscultate in the 4 main areas for heart sounds using diaphragm part of the stethoscope, ensure to palpate carotid pulse simultaneously, to ensure each beat is corresponding correctly. Count down from sternal edge (Angle of Louis). State that you would listen in with the diaphragm part of the stethoscope and then the bell.

- Aortic Valve – 2nd ICS to the right
- Pulmonic Valve – 2nd ICS to the left
- Mitral Valve – 5th ICS midclavicular
- Tricuspid Valve – 4th ICS Parasternal edge

Special tests for murmurs:
Ejection systolic murmur (ESM) – aortic stenosis: Ask the patient to hold their breath while you auscultate the carotid pulse, so you can listen for the radiate of the ESM. Use the diaphragm part of your stethoscope.

Aortic regurgitation: ask the patient to sit forward and auscultate over the aortic arch – the left side. During expiration an early diastolic murmur may be heard (ask patient to breathe in and out). Use the diaphragm part of your stethoscope.

Pansystolic murmurs/mitral regurgitation: ask patient to roll onto left side and auscultate over the mitral area during expiration (ask patient to breath in and out). Note that a pansystolic murmur can radiate to the axilla. Use the diaphragm part of your stethoscope.

Mitral stenosis: while still lying on left side, use the bell side of the stethoscope to check for a mid-diastolic murmur.

The bell is used for frequency sounds
The diaphragm is used for high frequency sounds

Abdomen: get on knees, to observe from the same level. Check for abdominal aortic aneurysm- so expansible VS pulsatile. You can also mention that you can listen for any renal bruits.

Take the femoral pulse – remember to inform the patient of this beforehand. Mention that you can check for radio-femoral delay at this point. Remember the pulse is located between the anterior superior Iliac spine and the pubic symphysis.

Lung auscultation: auscultate over the lower lung bases, listen out for coarse crackles and air entry.

Coarse crackles will indicate pulmonary oedema which is associated with left sided ventricular failure.

Absent air entry maybe be suggestive of pleural effusion caused by left ventricular.

At this point, palpate for any sacral oedema- check for pitting oedema.

Legs: inspect the legs for any obvious scars, ulcers (any evidence of peripheral arterial disease) any obvious pitting peripheral oedema- check thing my pressing finger over ankle for at least 10 seconds. Take the Popliteal pulse, posterior tibial pulse and the dorsalis pedis pulse on both sides.

4 To Complete

Summarise findings in logical and structured manner

Offer appropriate diagnosis and differential diagnoses if appropriate

Further investigations/examinations: peripheral vascular examination, respiratory examination, measure blood pressure, record a 12-lead ECG, bloods.

Thank the patient

Wash hands

PERIPHERAL VASCULAR EXAM

1 ICE – Introduction, Consent and Exposure

Introduce yourself: full name and your role

Confirm patient identity (name and date of birth)

Consent for examination

Explain the examination: explain what you will be doing, so looking at hands face, chest and legs, listening to the heart and checking pulses around the body

Appropriate position and exposure: 45° and expose chest (NB DO NOT use the word 'expose'). You can say 'I will need you to remove all clothing (including your bra) from waist upwards.' Also will need to remove clothing away from lower legs.

Always ask about chaperone

Wash/gel hands

Always check for pain before starting, acknowledge pain and say, 'I can see you are in pain, hopefully we can get you sorted,' Ask if they would like any pain relief and say you will arrange for some after the examination.

2 General Inspection

Patient: in pain, pallor, short of breath, obvious scars, peripheral oedema, body habitus, age

Surroundings: oxygen masks, IV drips, ECG/heart monitors

3 Examination

Hands: clubbing – ask them to do Schamroth's window, peripheral cyanosis, tendon xanthoma- hyperlipidaemia, and check for capillary refill – count out loud for 5 seconds and mention capillary refill return time. Check for tar staining, any skin colour changes (mottled, pale or pink). Assess the temperature of the hands.

Wrists: record the radial pulse (time for 15 seconds and then multiply number by 4) comment on the rate, rhythm, volume. Check for radio-radial delay, and mention you can also check for radio- femoral delay – sign for aortic coarctation

Arms: take both brachial pulses – comment on rate, rhythm and volume.

Offer to check blood pressure in both arms, if there is a difference of more than 10mmHg this would be of significance.

Eyes: corneal arcus (can be normal finding in over 50s, otherwise consider hyperlipidaemia) xanthelasma – also a sign of hyperlipidaemia, conjunctival pallor – sign of anaemia.

Mouth: check for central cyanosis and for angular stomatitis on the corners of the mouth – sign of iron deficiency.

Neck: take the carotid pulse, one at a time, as bilateral palpation of carotid pulses simultaneously can compromise the arterial blood flow to the brain and stimulate the vagus nerve leading to vagal syncope. (Comment on rate, rhythm, volume). Also assess JVP.

Abdomen: get on knees, to observe from the same level, note any colour changes such as grey turners which is found around the flanks and cullens which is bruising around the umbilicus. Check for abdominal aortic aneurysm- so expansible VS pulsatile. You can also mention that you can listen for any renal bruits. Palpate all 9 regions.

Take the femoral pulse – remember to inform the patient of this beforehand. Mention that you can check for radio-femoral delay at this point. Remember the pulse is located between the anterior superior iliac spine and the pubic symphysis.

Aortic dissection – Radio-radial delay

Aortic coarctation – Radio-femoral delay

Lower limb: before starting always check if in any pain

1. Inspection of the legs
   - Skin colour changes (mottled or pale)
   - Ischaemia changes
   - Trophic changes (shiny, hair loss, any ulcers)
   - Ankle oedema/swelling
   - Muscle wasting
   - Any obvious scars i.e. from CABG
   - Check for varicose veins
   - Check in between toes and heel
   - Don't forget the 6 P's – pallor, painful, pulseless, perishingly cold, paraesthesia, paralysis.

2. Palpation of legs
   - Temperature, ensure to check bilaterally
   - Capillary refill
   - Palpate all lower pulse: popliteal, posterior tibial, dorsalis pedis pulses.
   - Squeeze calves to check for critical ischaemia

- Assess sensation with fine touch, or even with monofilament, check vibration sensation

3. Special test: Buerger's angle
   - This is to assess the filling and reperfusion times
   - Before starting always check if patient is in pain
   - Ask patient to lie supine and lift their legs until the heel becomes pale – say you would hold for 30 seconds, if the legs don't become pale – then test is normal
   - If it does become pale, this is a positive test
   - Then ask patient to sit and let legs hang over the edge of the bed and say you would observe for 2–3 minutes. If the legs become pale and then red this is a positive test and implies significant peripheral arterial disease. (Pallor -> reactive hyperaemia (rubor))

4 To Complete

Summarise findings in logical and structured manner

Offer appropriate diagnosis and differential diagnoses if appropriate

Further investigations/examinations: cardiovascular examination, measure blood pressure, record a 12-lead ECG, bloods, Doppler ultrasound for pulses and ankle brachial pulse index

Thank the patient

Wash hands

Ankle Brachial Pulse Index – ABPI

Intermittent claudication	<0.9 ABPI
Acute ischaemia	ABPI <0.6 and 6 Ps
Critical ischaemia	Tissue loss and rest pain. ABPI <0.3

Types of Ulcers

Venous ulcers	Superficial, irregular, gaiter area
Arterial ulcers	Deep, punched out, clear borders, distal – toes
Mixed	Venous and arterial picture
Neuropathic	Over pressure points – heels, back of heels. Punched out, deep, loss of sensation

RESPIRATORY EXAMINATION

1 ICE – Introduction, Consent and Exposure

Introduce yourself: full name and your role

Confirm patient identity (name and date of birth)

Consent for examination

Explain the examination: explain what you will be doing, so looking at hands face, chest and legs, listening to the heart and checking pulses around the body

Appropriate position and exposure: 45 ° and expose chest (NB DO NOT use the word 'expose'). You can say, 'I will need you to remove all clothing (including your bra) from waist upwards'. Also will need to remove clothing away from lower legs.

Always ask about chaperone

Wash/gel hands

Always check for pain before starting, acknowledge pain and say, 'I can see you are in pain, hopefully we can get you sorted.' Ask if they would like any pain relief and say you will arrange for some after the examination.

2 General Inspection

Patient: in pain, pallor, short of breath, obvious scars, peripheral oedema, obvious cough or wheeze/stridor, cachexia, central cyanosis

Surroundings: oxygen masks, IV drips, ECG/heart monitors, sputum pot

3 Examination

Hands: Any peripheral cyanosis which may suggest hypoxaemia, tar staining, check capillary refill, temperature, check for clubbing – suggestive of lung disease, cystic fibrosis, interstitial lung disease and bronchiectasis.

Check for tremor:
Fine tremor: ask patient to hold both hands out in front of them – fine tremor may be caused by overuse of salbutamol.

Flapping tremor – ASTERIX – Ask the patient to stretch their hands out in front of them and cock their wrists back (state you would hold them in that position for 30 seconds). Observe for Asterix – this is caused by the irregular lapses of posture causing a flapping of the hands. The underlying cause can be CO_2 retention due to type 2 respiratory failure i.e. COPD. There are also other causes such as hepatic encephalopathy.

Take the radial pulse:

Pulse abnormalities caused by respiratory disease:

Bounding pulse – this can be associated type 2 respiratory failure – CO_2 retention

Pulsus paradoxus- when the pulse decreases during inspiration – this can be a sign of severe asthma and COPD exacerbations.

Take the respiratory rate:

While taking the pulse do this, so the patient doesn't become aware and conscious of their breathing as this can give false readings.

Normal range (12-20)

Neck: you can mention that you can measure the JVP, but won't have to do it; a raised JVP can be due to pulmonary hypertension.

Tracheal position: assess the tracheal position, ensure to inform patient before doing this, use your index finger and place into the thorax. Mention any difference which can be caused by tracheal deviation caused by tension pneumothorax – the trachea will deviate towards the lobar collapse.

Cricosternal distance: this is the difference between the inferior border of the cricoid cartilage and suprasternal notch. Normal is between 3–4 fingers. If extended this can be due to hyperinflation of the lungs caused by asthma or COPD.

Lymph nodes: do this from behind if possible, starting from submental area to occipital nodes

Face: pallor, plethoric complexion – this may be due to CO2 retention, central cyanosis

Chest inspection: obvious scars, chest wall deformities such as pectus excavatum or pectus carinatum, hyperinflated chest, barrel chest

Chest palpation: check for chest expansion by placing hands on chest and observing the thumbs move in a symmetrical pattern in normal breathing.

Chest percussion: percuss all the major areas of the chest wall and note the different changes in sound, such as resonance, hyperresonance, dullness and stony dullness. Note to always compare with opposite side.

Resonance	Normal finding
Hyperresonance	Pneumothorax
Dullness	Consolidation/pulmonary oedema
Stony dullness	Pleural effusion

Chest auscultation: all over the major areas of chest wall, note on bilateral equal air entry. Note any obvious lung sounds such as crackles – fine or coarse, wheeze. Listen for heart sounds at this point too. Note to always compare with opposite side.

Special tests:

Vocal resonance: auscultate over major areas of chest wall while the patient is repeating '111' in a low voice/tone.

Tactile vocal fremitus: this is done by placing hands on patient's chest wall while they say '99'.

Both tests are assessing the conduction of the sound going through lung tissue.

Posterior chest: always assess the posterior side, completing the inspection, palpation, percussion and auscultation. At this point check for any sacral oedema.

Legs: assess the legs for any peripheral oedema, ensure to check for pitting oedema by holding for 10 seconds. Assess the colour, temperature. Look for any signs of a DVT – any swelling, compare both legs. Look for any obvious scars.

4 To Complete

Summarise findings in logical and structured manner

Offer appropriate diagnosis and differential diagnoses if appropriate

Further investigations/examinations: cardiovascular examination, check oxygen saturation and other vital signs, peak flow, chest x-ray, ABG (Remember BOXES).

Thank the patient

Wash hands

DIABETIC FOOT EXAMINATION

1 ICE – Introduction, Consent and Exposure

Introduce yourself: full name and your role

Confirm patient identity (name and date of birth)

Consent for examination

Explain the examination: explain what you will be doing, so will be doing a diabetic foot check, which will involve having a thorough look at both feet, checking sensation, reflexes and checking the pulses in the feet.

Appropriate position and exposure: shoes and socks off (NB DO NOT use the word 'expose').

Always ask about chaperone

Wash/gel hands

Always check for pain before starting, acknowledge pain and say, 'I can see you are in pain, hopefully we can get you sorted.' Ask if they would like any pain relief and say you will arrange for some after the examination.

Gather your equipment

Monofilament

Tendon hammer

Tuning fork 128 Hz

2 General Inspection

Patient: in pain, pallor, gait

Surroundings: walking aids, medication, patient's footwear

3 Gait

Ask the patient to walk across the room and assess their gait. Ask them to let you know if they feel any discomfort or pain.

Assess
- speed
- steps
- turning
- stance

Types of gait in diabetic patients

- abnormal gait caused by peripheral neuropathy
- conservative gait caused by the walking speed reduced and stance broadened.
- high- stepping gait caused by foot droop

4 Inspection of the Feet (NB the IPPA model – Inspection, Palpation, Percussion and Auscultation)

When inspecting the feet, ensure to compare both sides, check in between web spaces, the toe nails, the heels and soles of the feet (do this for every part).

Look for peripheral cyanosis, any pallor, colour changes, any ulcers (arterial or venous) gangrene, amputations, scars, corns, calluses, skin thickening, dryness.

Types of ulcers

Venous ulcers	Superficial, irregular, gaiter area
Arterial ulcers	Deep, punched out, clear borders, distal – toes
Mixed	Venous and arterial picture
Neuropathic	Over pressure points – heels, back of heels. Punched out, deep, loss of sensation

5 Palpation

Assess the temperature using the dorsal aspect of your hand, start from mid shin of the legs and work your way down.

Check pulses: palpate the posterior tibial and dorsalis pedis pulse, do this bilaterally (NB ensure the correct location of the pulses)

Dorsalis pedis: lateral to the extensor hallucis longus tendon (you can ask patient to raise their big toe to make palpation easier)

Posterior tibial: 2cm below and behind the medial malleolus

6 Sensation

Using the monofilament, always demonstrate how this will feel on a central part of the patient's body i.e. the sternum.

Explain to the patient that you will be checking the sensation in their feet using this. You will need them to close their eyes, and you will tap them with this equipment in various places. Ask them to let you know every time they feel the monofilament by saying 'yes'.

You will press the monofilament against the skin until it bends slightly

Areas to check:

- The pulp of the hallux and all 5 digits
- The metatarsophalangeal joints – 1,3 and 5
- Check at least in 5 areas and bilaterally
- Anything above 70% felt is normal

7 Vibration Sensation

You will check this using the 128Hz tuning fork. Again you show the patient before on a central part of the body. Explain to the patients that you will need them to close their eyes and you place this equipment on various parts of the feet, they should tell you when they can feel it vibrating and when it stops

- Tap the tuning fork and place on the interphalangeal joint of the big toe. If the patient says they can feel that, you do not need to assess further. However, if the sensation is impaired at this point, go on to assessing the more proximal joints such as the metatarsal joint of the big toe -> ankle joint -> knee joint.

8 Proprioception

- This is to assess the joint position Again, explain to the patient what you will be doing.
- Start at the interphalangeal joint of the big toe – hold the distal phalanx of the big toe by its side (because if you hold the nail bed, this can allow the patient to know which direction, based on the pressure) – demonstrate the movements up and down
- Ask the patient to close their eyes and tell them to tell you when you are moving up or down
- Do this at least 3 times

9 Reflexes

You will need to assess the ankle reflex.

There are two ways to check this:

1. Ask patient to slightly abduct their hip when lying, flex their knee and dorsiflex the ankle, then tap the Achilles tendon with the tendon hammer. You will be observing for the contraction in the gastrocnemius muscle.
2. Ask patient to kneel on a chair, holding onto it, and tap the Achilles tendon.

10 To Complete

Summarise findings in logical and structured manner

Offer appropriate diagnosis and differential diagnoses if appropriate

Further investigations/examinations: cardiovascular examination, peripheral vascular examination, doppler, HbA1c bloods, capillary blood glucose

Thank the patient

Wash hands

NEUROLOGICAL EYE EXAMINATION

Assessing cranial nerves 2, 3, 4 and 6

1 ICE – Introduction, Consent and Exposure

Introduce yourself: full name and your role

Confirm patient identity (name and date of birth)

Consent for examination

Explain the examination: explain you will be doing an examination of the eyes and will also need to come quite close to have a look at the back of the eye using special equipment

Appropriate position and exposure: patient to sit in a chair.

Always ask about chaperone

Wash/gel hands

Always check for pain before starting, acknowledge pain and say, 'I can see you are in pain, hopefully we can get you sorted.' Ask if they would like any pain relief and say you will arrange for some after the examination.

2 General Inspection

Patient's health: do they wear glasses, eye patches, eye drops?

The eyes: scars, swelling, discharge, obvious foreign body, obvious infection, redness

3 Visual Acuity

You will need a Snellen chart for this, which should be provided, but always check the distance is correct – the preferable distance is 6 metres.

- Ask the patient to cover one eye at a time and start reading the chart from the lowest line and work their way up if they are unable to read the lowest line
- If the patient can read the lowest line this means their visual acuity is 6/6 or 20/20
- Ensure to do one eye at a time
- You can mention that at this point you can assess the patient's near vision using a fine print to read

4 Visual Fields

This is to compare the patient's visual field with your own. You will need to sit opposite the patient, with a 1-metre distance.

- Ask the patient to cover one eye with their hand
- If the patient covers their left, you should cover your right (mirroring your patient)
- Ask the patient to focus on your nose and not move their head or eyes at any point during this
- Start from the periphery and slowly move the target towards the centre, so you will be moving your fingers, and ask the patient to let you know as soon as they see your fingers
- The process needs to be done for each of the visual quadrants and then do the same for the other eye

If the patient can't see the fingers, this may be suggestive of reduced visual fields.

Types of visual field defects:

Bitemporal hemianopia: this is the loss of the temporal visual field in both eyes, resulting in tunnel vision. This usually occurs if there is a compression of the optic chiasm by tumour (e.g. pituitary adenoma).

Homonymous field defects: this affects the same side of the visual field in each eye. This is usually caused by strokes, tumours, etc. so anything that is affecting the visual pathways posterior to the optic chiasm.

Hemianopias: if half the vision is affected

Quadrantanopias: if a quarter of the vision is affected

5 Pupillary Reflexes

Direct pupillary reflex:

Shine the light using a pen torch into the patient's pupil and observe for the pupillary restriction in the ipsilateral eye.

Normal direct pupillary reflex will involve the constriction of the pupil that the light is being shone into (check both eyes).

Consensual pupillary reflex:

Shine the light using a pen torch into the patient's same pupil, but this time look out for the pupillary restriction in the contralateral eye.

Swinging eye test:

Move the pen torch rapidly in between both eyes to check – observe for the dilatation of the pupil

Accommodation reflex: ask the patient to focus on something behind you, then Place your finger about 20cm away from their face and ask them to look at your finger and then back at the other focus point and then bring your finger closer and ask the patient to look at them again. Observe for the constriction and convergence bilaterally.

6 Eye Movements

Ask the patient to keep their head still whilst following your finger with their eyes. Ask them to inform you if they feel any pain in their eyes or see double at any point. Move your finger slowly in an H pattern. You will observe for any restriction of movements of the eye and nystagmus.

Abnormalities of the eye movements may be due to cranial nerve palsies such as oculomotor, trochlear, abducens and vestibular nerve pathology.

7 Ophthalmoscopy or Fundoscopy

Explain what you will be doing: you will be using a piece of equipment which will allow you to look at the back of their eyes. In order to do this, you have to make the room dark and will have to come quite close and you may need to place your hands on their forehead so you don't bump into one another.

Key point: even if you cannot darken the room, always mention this to the examiner

- Set the ophthalmoscope to your visual acuity
- Assess the red reflex – look through the ophthalmoscope, shine the light towards the patient's eye from a distance and observe the red reflex in each pupil. (this is caused by the light reflecting from the vascularised retina)

Absent red reflex: cataracts are main causes in adults, others include vitreous haemorrhage and retinal detachment. In children, usually due to retinoblastoma or vitreous haemorrhage.

- Assess the fundus and optic disc: assess one eye at a time. Start with, say, the patient's right eye, then you should hold the ophthalmoscope with your right hand and vice versa. Place your other hand on patient's forehead to prevent bumping into one another. Come in from a 45-degree angle and move in slowly, try find a blood vessel and follow that through to the optic disc.

The Optic Disc – 3 Cs:

Colour: healthy optic disc should appear to be a pink-orange with a pale centre.

Contour: it should be clear and well defined. If there is swelling this may be suggestive of papilledema which is secondary to raised intracranial pressure.

Cup: the cup is pale centre and there should be a cup-disc ratio of 0.3.

Ensure to assess both eyes.

8 Questions

You may be shown pictures of some changes

Diabetic eye changes

- Background retinopathy – scattered haemorrhages described as 'dot and blot' haemorrhages. Hard and soft exudates, not affecting macula and non-sight threatening.
- Diabetic maculopathy – haemorrhages and hard exudates within macula. Leakage of fluid from vasculature and macula oedema. Treated with focal laser.
- Pre-proliferative retinopathy – more than 5 cotton wool spots, venous changes include thickening and beading. This indicates retinal ischaemia. Can be sight threatening.
- Proliferative retinopathy – new vessels forming, these new blood vessels can bleed causing 'vitreous haemorrhage'. This will require extensive laser treatment.

Hypertensive retinopathy

- Grade 1 – vascular attenuation, blood vessel walls get thickened.
- Grade 2 – irregularly located tight constrictions 'AV nicking/nipping'. Salus's sign– thickened, hardened artery crosses a vein
- Grade 3 – retinal oedema, cotton wool spots (soft exudate) due to ischaemia and flame shaped haemorrhages – 'Copper wiring'
- Grade 4 – optic disc oedema and macular star – 'silver wiring'

Papilledema

- Optic disc swelling caused due to raised intracranial pressure, maybe due to a tumour, haemorrhage (subdural, extradural or subarachnoid), increased cerebrospinal fluid (CSF)
- Usually bilateral and occurs over a period of time – hours to weeks
- Unilateral presentations are RARE
- Disc will appear pinkish and not pale and will be swollen towards you

9 To Complete

Summarise findings in logical and structured manner

Offer appropriate diagnosis and differential diagnoses if appropriate

Further investigations/examinations: cranial nerve examination, HbA1c bloods, capillary blood glucose, measure blood pressure

Thank the patient

Wash hands

CRANIAL NERVE EXAMINATION

Cranial Nerve Number	Cranial Nerve	Nerve Type	Function
1	Olfactory	Sensory	Smell
2	Optic	Sensory	Vision
3	Oculomotor	Motor	Most eye movements
4	Trochlear	Motor	Moves eyes
5	Trigeminal	Sensory & Motor	Face sensation, mastication
6	Abducens	Motor	Abducts eye
7	Facial	Sensory & Motor	Facial expression/taste
8	Vestibulocochlear	Sensory	Hearing, balance
9	Glossopharyngeal	Sensory & Motor	Taste, gag reflex
10	Vagus	Sensory & Motor	Gag reflex
11	Accessory	Motor	Shoulder shrug
12	Hypoglossal	Motor	Swallowing & speech

1 ICE – Introduction, Consent and Exposure

Introduce yourself: full name and your role

Confirm patient identity (name and date of birth)

Consent for examination

Explain the examination: 'I would like to assess the nerves in your face, which is part of the neurological assessment.'

Appropriate position and exposure: patient to sit in a chair about 1–2 metres away

Always ask about chaperone

Wash/gel hands

2 General Inspection

Patient's health, any obvious facial droop, drooping of eyelid, in obvious pain

3 Examination

Olfactory (CN 1): ask the patient if they have noticed any changes in their sense. (NB this isn't routinely tested but you can mention that you can test this with coffee or lemon). The sense of smell can be affected by trauma, frontal lobe tumour, meningitis.

Optic, oculomotor, trochlear and abducens (CN 2, 3, 4 & 6) (note 2,3,4 and 6th cranial nerve should be assessed together).

Visual acuity

You will need a Snellen chart for this, which should be provided, but always check the distance is correct. The preferable distance is 6 metres.

- Ask the patient to cover one eye at a time and start reading the chart from the lowest line and work their way up if they are unable to read the lowest line
- If the patient can read the lowest line this means their visual acuity is 6/6 or 20/20
- Ensure to do one eye at a time
- You can mention that at this point you can assess the patient's near vision using a fine print to read

Visual fields

This is to compare the patient's visual field with your own. You will need to sit opposite the patient, with a 1-metre distance.

- Ask the patient to cover one eye with their hand
- If the patient covers their left, you should cover your right (mirroring your patient)
- Ask the patient to focus on your nose and not move their head or eyes at any point during this
- Start from the periphery and slowly move the target towards the centre, so you will be moving your fingers, and you ask the patient to let you know as soon as they see your fingers.
- The process needs to be done for each of the visual quadrants and then do the same for the other eye.

Pupillary reflexes

- **Direct pupillary reflex:**

Shine the light using a pen torch into the patient's pupil and observe for the pupillary restriction in the ipsilateral eye. Normal direct pupillary reflex will involve the constriction of the pupil that the light is being shone into (Check both eyes).

- **Consensual pupillary reflex:**

Shine the light using a pen torch into the patient's same pupil, but this time look out for the pupillary restriction in the contralateral eye.

- **Swinging eye test:**

Move the pen torch rapidly in between both eyes to check – observe for the dilatation of the pupil.

- **Accommodation reflex:**

Ask the patient to focus on something behind you, then place your finger about 20cm away from their face and ask them to look at your finger and then back at the other focus point and then bring your finger closer and ask the patient to look at them again. Observe for the constriction and convergence bilaterally.

Eye movements

- Ask the patient to keep their head still whilst following your finger with their eyes. Ask them to inform you if they feel any pain in their eyes or see double at any point. Move your finger slowly in an H pattern. You will observe for any restriction of movements of the eye and nystagmus.
- Abnormalities of the eye movements may be due to cranial nerve palsies such as oculomotor, trochlear, abducens and vestibular nerve pathology.

Trigeminal (CN 5)

Sensory: ask patient to close their eyes, 'Say yes when you feel me tapping your face'. Check opposite sides of the face, comparing one side to the other. Ask patient to let you know if it feels the same on both sides. Assess both fine and pain touch.

The 3 divisions to check:

1. Ophthalmic – above eyebrows
2. Maxillary- over zygoma
3. Mandibular- chin, either side of midline

Motor: ask the patient to open jaw against resistance. Push against and upwards on the patient's chin and say, 'Open jaw against my hand'. The jaw will deviate on the side of the weakness -> Pterygoid muscle.

Ask patient to clench their jaw and palpate for the masseter muscle contraction above the angle of the jaw.

Reflexes: (not usually done in OSCES, but mention it)
Corneal reflex – using cotton wool
Jaw reflex – not routinely assessed

Facial (CN 7)
Inspect: facial symmetry
Motor: ask the patient to do the following:

- Raise eyebrows
- Scrunch eyes and ask them to resist you from opening the eyes
- Purse lips together
- Smile and show your teeth
- Puff out cheeks and try to push the air out using your hands

Any weakness shown here may suggest an upper motor neuron defect such as a stroke.

Vestibulocochlear (CN 8)

- Crude hearing test: ask the patient to cover one ear at a time and whisper a number into the uncovered ear, ask them to repeat that number to you. Repeat this in both ears.
- Rinne's test: use a 512Hz tuning fork to check this. Tap the tuning fork in your hands and place the round base on the mastoid process. Ask your patient to let you know when the sound stops. Then lift the fork and place the long ends near the patients' ear. Now ask if they can hear it again. Do this on both sides. You are checking the air to bone conduction. The air conduction should be louder than bone conduction. You can ask the patient which was louder. If they can't hear it again then there is a deficit in that ear.
- Weber's test: use a 512Hz tuning fork for this test also. Tap the tuning fork and place the round base on the patient's forehead between their eyes. Ask them to let you know which side they can hear it louder. It should be the same on both sides

but if one side is louder than the other this can be suggestive of that side having a conductive deficit, or the contralateral side has a sensorineural deficit.

Glossopharyngeal and Vagus (CN 9 & 10)

- **Inspect:** ask the patient to open their mouth and say 'ahh'. Using your pen torch you will inspect the symmetry of the palate (CN 9) and check for uvula deviation (CN 10) – this will deviate away from the lesion
- **Motor:** ask the patient to cough and swallow and assess their speech
- **Gag reflex:** this isn't routinely checked, but mention that you can do this

Accessory (CN 11)

Inspect: check for any trapezius or sternocleidomastoid muscle wasting

Motor: ask the patient to shrug their shoulders while you resist – testing the trapezius muscle – and then ask the patient to turn their head to one side at a time against resistance. This is testing the contralateral sternocleidomastoid muscle.

Hypoglossal (CN 12)

Inspect: inspect the tongue, look for any muscle wasting or fasciculations which can be caused by lower motor neuron lesions i.e. bulbar palsy.

Motor: ask the patient to stick their tongue out and move side to side. Ask the patient to push into cheeks and check power by resisting.

4 To Complete

- Summarise findings in logical and structured manner
- Offer appropriate diagnosis and differential diagnoses if appropriate
- Further investigations/examinations: upper and lower limb neurological examination, cerebellar examination, CT/MRI scans, bloods
- Thank the patient
- Wash hands

UPPER LIMB NEUROLOGICAL EXAMINATION

Key

UMN – upper motor neuron
LMN – lower motor neuron

1 ICE – Introduction, Consent and Exposure

Introduce yourself: full name and your role

Confirm patient identity (name and date of birth)

Consent for examination

Explain the examination: 'I would like to do an upper limb neurological exam, which will involve examining your hands and arms mainly, and I will be checking the tone, power, coordination, sensation and reflexes.'

Appropriate position and exposure: patient's upper body. They can leave bra on, sitting up on the couch

Always ask about chaperone

Wash/gel hands

2 General Inspection

Patient: is the patient well, in pain, SWIFT (using SWIFT will make sure you don't miss anything out)

S   Scars/skin – neurofibromas, café au lait spots

W Wasting of muscles, general wasting or thenar or hypothenar wasting (UMN)

I   Involuntary movements

F   Fasciculations (LMN)

T   Tremors

Around the bed: walking aids, medication, oxygen

TOPCARS (A good way to remember all the assessments of a neurological examination)

T TONE, P POWER, C COORDINATION, R REFLEXES and S SENSATION

3 Examination (always check for any pain before starting)

TONE

UMN: tone is increased

LMN: tone is decreased

Parkinson's: cogwheel rigidity

Pronator drift: ask the patient to extend arms out in front of them with their palms facing upwards and then ask them to close their eyes. If there is a pronator drift this can suggest pyramidal weakness. If there is an upwards drift this can suggest cerebellar lesion. The upwards drift can be further accentuated by pushing down on the patient's wrists briskly and letting go quickly (REBOUND).

Tone: (you can do all these movements in one go)

- Elbow: hold the patient's hand in a hand shaking position, support their elbow with your other hand and then flex and extend their elbow to full range repeatedly.
- Forearm: again, in the same position as above, but keep their elbows at 90 degrees and then pronate and supinate their hand in alternating directions. Do this repeatedly.
- Wrist: hold the patient's forearm, just proximal to their wrist and then flex, extend and rotate their hand on their wrist.

POWER (ensure you know your Dermatomes)

Assess one side at a time, so you can compare one side to the other. Support the side that is being tested. Grade the power against the MRC grading 0–5

0   nothing
1   flicker of muscle contraction
2   gravity eliminated
3   gravity
4   some resistance
5   full power

Show the patient the movements when explaining

- **Shoulder abduction (C5):** patient abducts shoulders and raises arm to horizontal plane. To check resistance – push down. 'Don't let me push your arms down.'
- **Elbow flexion (C6):** ask patient to bring arms in a sagittal plane towards body, with elbows being flexed. Support the ipsilateral elbow with one hand and try to pull the wrist away (show them.) 'Put your arms out like this, like you are boxing, I am going to pull your wrist away, don't let me.'

- **Elbow extension (C7):** same position as above but try and push their wrist towards them. 'Push me away while I hold your wrist.'
- **Wrist extension (C7):** ask patient to hold out their arms straight while making fists. Hold the ipsilateral wrist with one hand and using the other push their wrist down. 'Hold your fists out like this, I will push your fists down, don't let me.'
- **Finger extension (C7):** ask patient to hold out their arms straight with their fingers extended. Hold the ipsilateral metacarpals with one hand and use the other hand to push down their fingers. 'Hold your fingers straight out like this, I will push your finger down, don't let me.'
- **Finger flexion (C8):** interlock grips with the patient and try to open their fingers. 'Grip my finger and don't let me pull out.'
- **Finger abduction (T1):** ask the patient to spread their fingers out. Push their little and index fingers inwards. 'Spread your fingers out and don't let me push them in.'
- **Thumb abduction (T1):** ask the patient to point their thumbs towards the ceiling and push their thumbs down. 'Don't let me push your thumbs down.'

COORDINATION

Finger to nose test: ask the patient to hold their index finger out. Using your index finger touch theirs. Ask the patient to keep their head still and touch your finger and their nose in between (alternate between finger and nose). Ask them to do this as fast as they can. Repeat on both sides. Intention tremor and past pointing can be suggestive of cerebellar lesions i.e. dysmetria caused by a cerebellar lesion.

Dysdiadochokinesia: ask the patient to hold one palm up and clap into the other hand repeatedly but ask them to flip the hand when hitting the palm, so top bottom top... do this on both sides.

Impaired coordination may be suggestive of dysdiadochokinesia caused by a cerebellar lesion.

REFLEXES

Check reflexes using the tendon hammer. Hold the tendon hammer at the end of the stick and do a pendulum swing. If a reflex is not elicited, make sure the patient is relaxed and give them a distraction such as 'grit your teeth'. Check both sides.

Types of reflexes:

Normal, brisk, absent or reduced

- **Biceps (C5/6):** ask the patient to relax their arm across their lap. Ask them to relax. Place your index finger over the biceps tendon and then strike onto your finger.
- **Triceps (C7):** hold their ipsilateral wrist with one hand, ask them to let their hand go floppy. Strike the triceps tendon.

- **Supinator (C4/6):** ask the patient to relax across their lap, place your index and middle finger over the brachioradialis tendon and strike your fingers.

SENSATION

This is broken down into 4 parts:

Fine/light sensation (dorsal)

Pain (spinothalamic) sensation

Proprioception (spinothalamic)

Vibration sensation (dorsal)

For the sensations, before starting always show the patient how it will feel on a central part of the body first i.e. sternum. Start from distal to proximal.

Sensation pathologies:

Glove and stockings – distal loss. Common finding in diabetics.

Fine/light touch: use a cotton wool and ask the patient to close their eyes and to let you know when they can feel you tapping them with the cotton wool. Ensure to compare one side to the other. Start from C4 – C5 – C6 – C7 – C8 – T1 – T2.

Pain sensation: use a neurological pin and ask the patient to close their eyes and to let you know when they can feel you tapping them with the pin. Ensure to compare one side to the other. Start from C4 – C5 – C6 – C7 – C8 – T1 – T2.

Proprioception: hold the proximal phalanx of the thumb using your index finger and thumb. Use your other hand to hold each side of the distal phalanx. Show the patient up and down positions and then ask them to close their eyes. Move their thumb up and down, do this at least 3 times, ask the patient to tell you which direction you are moving their thumb in.

Vibration: you will check this using the 128Hz tuning fork. Again you show the patient first on a central part of the body. Explain to the patient that you will need them to close their eyes and you place this equipment on their thumb; they should tell you when they can feel it vibrating and when it stops.

Tap the tuning fork and place on the interphalangeal joint of their thumb. If the patient says they can feel that, you do not need to assess further. However, if the sensation is impaired at this point, go on to assessing the more proximal joints such as the metacarpophalangeal joint and radial styloid, until they feel the vibration. Do this on both side

4 To Complete

- Temperature – you can check this by placing the tuning fork on the patient's sternum.
- Summarise findings in logical and structured manner
- Offer appropriate diagnosis and differential diagnoses if appropriate
- Further investigations/examinations: lower limb neurological examination, cranial nerve examination, cerebellar examination, CT/MRI scans, bloods
- Thank the patient
- Wash hands

UMN lesions	LMN lesions
Increased tone	Wasting and fasciculations
Spasticity	Decreased tone
Weakness	Weakness
Brisk reflexes, extensor plantar response	Reduced reflexes

LOWER LIMB NEUROLOGICAL EXAMINATION

1 ICE – Introduction, Consent and Exposure

Introduce yourself: full name and your role

Confirm patient identity (name and date of birth)

Consent for examination

Explain the examination: 'I would like to do a lower limb neurological exam, which will involve examining your legs and feet mainly, I will be checking the tone, power, coordination, sensation and reflexes.'

Appropriate position and exposure: undress lower half of the body, lying at 45 degrees on the couch.

Always ask about chaperone

Wash/gel hands

2 General Inspection

Patient: is the patient well, in pain, SWIFT (using SWIFT will make sure you don't miss anything out)

S Scars/skin – neurofibromas, café au lait spots
W Wasting of muscles, general wasting or thenar or hypothenar wasting (UMN)
I Involuntary movements
F Fasciculations (LMN)
T Tremors

Around the bed: walking aids, medication, oxygen

3 Gait

Ask the patient to do some normal walking across the room. 'Can you please walk to the door and back.'

Check heel to toe walking. Ataxia may be picked up, standing on toes and then heels; this tests distal power.

Types of gait

- Normal walking
- Hemiplegic (stroke patients)
- Spastic
- Foot drop
- Ataxic (broad)
- Myopathic waddling (Parkinsonian)

Do the Romberg's test – checking joint position sense:

TOPCARS (A good way to remember all the assessments of a neurological examination)

T TONE, P POWER, C COORDINATION, R REFLEXES AND S SENSATION

4 Examination (always check for any pain before starting)

TONE

Tone: ask the patient to relax their legs while lying. Tell them to let their legs go floppy and then roll each leg side to side, holding the leg by either side of their knee. Do this on both legs.

Spasticity: place one of your hands under the patient's knee and lift the leg briskly and let it drop gently.

Clonus: take the sole of the patient's foot in one hand and hold it up while holding the ipsilateral flexed knee in the other hand. Forcefully flex the ankle a few times and hold in a flexed firm position. Watch out for any involuntary rhythmic beats of the gastrocnemius contraction. More than 2 beats can be suggestive of an UMN lesion.

POWER

Assess one side at a time, so you can compare one side to the other. Support the side that is being tested. Grade the power against the MRC grading 0-5

0   nothing
1   flicker of muscle contraction
2   gravity eliminated
3   gravity
4   some resistance
5   full power

Show the patient the movements when explaining

- **Hip flexion (L2/L3):** ask the patient to lift their leg off the bed with their knee extended. Ensure to stabilise their contralateral hip with one hand and push down on the quadriceps just above the knee. 'Don't let me push your knee down.'
- **Hip extension (L4/L5):** while the leg is still lifted to about 30 degrees, stabilise the contralateral hip with one hand and hold under the patient's knee with the other hand. 'Push my hand down into the bed.'
- **Knee extension (L3/L4):** flex the patient's knee to about 90 degrees and stabilise their ipsilateral knee joint with one hand and hold the anterior side of the ankle with the other hand and push it towards them. 'Kick out your leg and don't let me push it towards you.'
- **Knee flexion (L5/S1):** same position as above but hold the posterior side of their ankle and pull it away. 'Pull your heel towards your bottom and don't let me pull it away.'
- **Ankle dorsiflexion (L4/L5):** ask the patient to straighten their leg and then dorsiflex their ankle, stabilise the ankle with one hand and using dorsal side of your other hand push the patient's foot down. 'Point your foot up towards you head and don't let me push it down.'
- **Ankle plantarflexion (S1/S2):** same position as above but have their ankle actively plantarflexed and pull it up with your fingers on the ball of the patient's foot. 'Point your foot down towards the bottom of the bed and don't let me push it down.'

Make sure to do this on both sides

COORDINATION

Heel to shin test: ask the patient to lift their opposite leg and touch their heel to their contralateral knee, and then bring the leg to their contralateral ankle. Then lift their leg and do it again, at least 3 times. Ensure to do both sides. If there is mal coordination this may suggest cerebellar disease.

REFLEXES

Check reflexes using the tendon hammer. Hold the tendon hammer at the end of the stick and do a pendulum swing. If a reflex is not elicited, make sure the patient is relaxed and give them a distraction such as 'grit your teeth'. Check both sides.

Types of reflexes:

Normal, brisk, absent or reduced

- **Knee (L3, L4):** have the knee in passive flexion, ask the patient to relax. While holding with your left wrist under the patient's knee, locate the tibial tuberosity and the inferior border of the patella, strike the patella in between.
- **Ankle (S1, S2):** Externally rotate the patient's ankle and flex their knee, so that their lower leg will be resting over their contralateral shin. Take their foot in your hand and gently passively dorsiflex their ankle. With the tendon hammer strike the Achilles tendon.
- **Plantar (Babinski response):** Explain to the patient that you will scrape the plantar surface of their foot using the other end of the tendon hammer. Start from the heel in a semi-circle and then around the lateral edge and to the ball of the big toe (toes curl in – normal response, if toes curl out – UMN lesion).

SENSATION

This is broken down into 4 parts:
Fine/light sensation (dorsal)
Pain (spinothalamic) sensation
Proprioception (spinothalamic)
Vibration sensation (dorsal)

For the sensations, before starting always show the patient how it will feel on a central part of the body first i.e. sternum. Start from distal to proximal.

Sensation pathologies:

Glove and stockings – distal loss. Common finding in diabetics.

Fine/light touch: use a cotton wool and ask the patient to close their eyes and to let you know when they can feel you tapping them with the cotton wool. Ensure to compare one side to the other. Start from L1-L2-L3-L4-L5-S1.

Pain sensation: use a neurological pin and ask the patient to close their eyes and to let you know when they can feel you tapping them with the pin. Ensure to compare one side to the other. Start from L1-L2-L3-L4-L5-S1.

Proprioception: hold the proximal phalanx of the big toe using your index finger and thumb. Use your other hand to hold each side of the distal phalanx. Show the patient up and down positions and then ask them to close their eyes. Move their thumb up and down, do this at least 3 times, ask the patient to tell you which direction you are moving their thumb in.

Vibration: you will check this using the 128Hz tuning fork, again you show the patient before on a central part of the body. Explain to the patient that you will need them to close their eyes and place this equipment on their thumb; they should tell you when they can feel it vibrating and when it stops.

- Tap the tuning fork and place on the interphalangeal joint of their big toe. If the patient says they can feel that, you do not need to assess further. However, if the sensation is impaired at this point, go on to assessing the more proximal joints such as the metatarsophalangeal joint, then medial malleolus and then tibial tuberosity, until they feel the vibration. Do this on both sides.

Temperature- you can mention you can check this by placing the tuning fork on the patient's sternum.

5 To Complete

- Summarise findings in logical and structured manner
- Offer appropriate diagnosis and differential diagnoses if appropriate
- Further investigations/examinations: upper limb neurological examination, cranial nerve examination, cerebellar examination, CT/MRI scans, bloods
- Thank the patient
- Wash hands

CEREBELLAR EXAMINATION

Case scenario: (NB the instructions for this may not be direct) A gentleman is describing tremor. Examine his gait and any other necessary examinations

1 ICE – Introduction, Consent and Exposure

Introduce yourself: full name and your role

Confirm patient identity (name and date of birth)

Consent for examination

Explain the examination: 'I understand you have a tremor so I would like to do a neurological examination, which will involve me checking how you walk, check your coordination and do some vision tests.'

Appropriate position and exposure: sitting in front of you

Always ask about chaperone

Wash/gel hands

2 General Inspection

Patient: is the patient well, in pain, SWIFT (using SWIFT will make sure you don't miss anything out)

S scars/skin – neurofibromas, café au lait spots
W wasting of muscles, general wasting or thenar or hypothenar wasting (UMN)
I involuntary movements
F Fasciculations (LMN)
T Tremors

Around the bed: walking aids, medication, oxygen, wheelchair, posture

3 Gait

Ask the patient to do some normal walking across the room 'can you please walk to the door and back'

Check heel to toe walking, ataxia may be picked up, standing on toes and then heels, this tests distal power

Types of gait

- Normal walking
- Hemiplegic (stroke patients)
- Spastic
- Foot drop
- Ataxic (broad)
- Myopathic waddling (parkinsonian)

Do the Romberg's test – checking joint position sense:

ATAXIA is a sign of cerebellar disease

Remember DANISH

D Dysdiadochokinesia and Dysmetria (past pointing)
A Ataxia
N Nystagmus
I Intention tremor
S Slurred or staccato speech
H Hypotonia

Causes of cerebellar disease:

- Multiple sclerosis
- Alcohol
- Vascular
- Inherited
- Space occupying lesion

4 Examination

Speech:

Assess their speech by asking them to say things like 'baby hippopotamus' or 'British constitution'. Watch out for any slurring, staccato speech (jerky speech)

Check that they can move their tongue from side to side

Face:

Do the H test to check eye movements, to check for the extraocular muscle function and pause at lateral gaze – look out for nystagmus

Upper limb:

Check the pronators drift; ask the patient to extend their arms out fully in front of them, note that an upwards drift may suggest cerebellar lesion.

You may check tone they will have reduced tone in cerebellar disease

Coordination:

- The finger nose test (intention tremor and dysmetria)
- Check for dysdiadochokinesia

Lower limb:

- Check tone in legs – hypotonia
- Coordination – heel to shin test

5 To Complete and Summarise findings in logical and structured manner

Offer appropriate diagnosis and differential diagnoses if appropriate

Further investigations/examinations: upper and lower limb neurological examination, cranial nerve examination, fundoscopy

Thank the patient

Wash hands

ENT – AUROSCOPY

1 ICE – Introduction, Consent and Exposure

Introduce yourself: full name and your role

Confirm patient identity (name and date of birth)

Consent for examination

Explain the examination: 'Today I would like to examine your ears; this will involve me having a look into your ears using a special equipment and I will also assess your hearing.'

Appropriate position and exposure: sitting in front of you

Always ask about chaperone

Wash/gel hands

Always check for pain before starting, acknowledge pain and say, 'I can see you are in pain, hopefully we can get you sorted.' Ask if they would like any pain relief and say you will arrange for some after the examination.

2 General Inspection

Patient: in pain, well

Surroundings: hearing aids, mobility aids, medication

3 Hearing Test

Start by asking the patient if they have noticed any recent changes in their hearing

- Crude hearing test: ask the patient to cover one ear at a time and whisper a number into the uncovered ear, then ask them to repeat that number to you. Repeat this in both ears.
- Rinne's test: use a 512Hz tuning fork to check this. Tap the tuning fork in your hands and place the round base on the mastoid process. Ask your patient to let you know when the sound stops. Then lift the fork and place the long ends near the patient's ear, now ask if they can hear it again. Do this on both sides. You are checking the air to bone conduction. The air conduction should be louder than bone conduction. You can ask the patient which was louder. If they can't hear it again then there is a deficit in that ear.

- Weber's test: use a 512Hz tuning fork for this test also. Tap the tuning fork and place the round base on the patient's forehead between their eyes. Ask them to let you know which side they can hear it louder. It should be the same on both sides but if one side is louder than the other this can be suggestive of that side having a conductive deficit, or the contralateral side has a sensorineural deficit.

4 Examination

Inspection:

Inspect the external ear section by section:

- Pinnae: asymmetry, deformity, piercing, scars, erythema, oedema, swelling, lesions
- Mastoid: erythema, swelling, scars
- Pre-auricular region: lymphadenopathy
- Any obvious discharge

Palpation:

- Palpate the external ear from tragus, helix, concha, mastoid and pinnae
- Palpate the pre-auricular and post auricular lymph nodes

Otoscopy:

Always start with the good ear first in patient who has pain or discomfort in one ear:

- Set the otoscope, attach a sterile speculum
- Pull the pinna up and back with your hand so you can straighten the external auditory canal
- The otoscope should be held in the right hand when assessing the right ear and vice versa. Hold the otoscope horizontally like a pencil, this will prevent damage to the ear in the case of a sudden movement.
- Assess both sides; once completed discard the speculum into a waste bin

What to comment on and look out for:

- Ear wax – ear wax impaction is a common cause for conductive hearing loss
- Erythema, oedema and discharge can be a cause of otitis extrena or perforation of the tympanic membrane
- Foreign body
- Assess the tympanic membrane which should appear as pearly grey and translucent, the same should be flat and non-bulging; if inflamed this can be due to otitis media.

- Check for light reflex 'cone of light'. This is the light reflected from the tympanic membrane; if there is an absence or distortion this can be associated with a bulging tympanic membrane caused by otitis media.
- Perforation – this can be caused by infection, cholesteatoma
- Scarring, usually caused due to repeated otitis media infections or after tympanostomy tube (Grommets)

5 To Complete

- Summarise findings in logical and structured manner
- Offer appropriate diagnosis and differential diagnoses if appropriate
- Further investigations/examinations: cranial nerve examination, formal hearing tests
- Thank the patient
- Wash hands

GASTROINTESTINAL EXAMINATION

1 ICE – Introduction, Consent and Exposure

Introduce yourself: full name and your role

Confirm patient identity (name and date of birth)

Consent for examination

Explain the examination: 'I would like to do a gastrointestinal examination; this will involve me examining your hands, face, tummy and legs.'

Appropriate position and exposure: sitting initially, then lying flat when examining abdomen. Remove all clothing from waist upwards.

Always ask about chaperone

Wash/gel hands

2 General Inspection

Patient: pain, pallor, vomiting, cachexia

Surroundings: vomit bowl, IV drip, medications

3 Examination

Hands

Nails: check for koilonychia (anaemia), Leukonychia (hypoalbuminemia), clubbing (malignancy)

Palmar: Palmar erythema, Dupentrens contracture

Dorsal: temperature and check for Asterix (hepatic encephalitis)

Face

Eyes: conjunctival pallor (anaemia), scleral Icterus (jaundice), Xanthelasma (hyperlipidaemia), Kayser- Fleischer rings (Wilson's disease)

Mouth: ulcers, aphthous ulcers, coeliac, glossitis (B12 Deficiency), angular stomatitis (anaemia), fetor hepaticus – foul odour caused by hepatic encephalitis, candidiasis

Neck

Mention you can check JVP

Examine all lymph nodes from submental – submandibular – pre-auricular – post auricular – anterior cervical chain – posterior cervical chain – occipital and supraclavicular region. Note the left supraclavicular lymphadenopathy is a sign of malignancy (Virchow's node)

Abdomen

Inspection: get to the same level of the abdomen, so on your knees, ensure patient is lying flat with their arms by their sides. Inspect for any obvious masses, scars, stomas, spider naevi (more than 5 is pathological), obvious distension, signs for pancreatitis, Cullen's sign (bruising and superficial oedema around the umbilicus) Grey Turner's (bruising of the flanks), gynaecomastia, hair loss

Palpation: start with light palpation, then deep palpation. Always check for pain before starting. If there is pain, start away from the pain and watch the patient as you palpate. Cover all 9 regions:

- Right upper quadrant (RUQ)
- Epigastric
- Left upper quadrant (LUQ)
- Right lumbar
- Umbilicus
- Left lumbar
- Right iliac fossa (RIF)

- Suprapubic
- Left iliac fossa (LIF)

Note any tenderness during palpation, any obvious masses, rebound tenderness, guarding.

Palpate the liver border: use one or both hands starting in the RIF using the edge of the hand. Ask the patient to take a deep breath and as they begin, palpate the abdomen. Feel for the liver edge pass below your hand during inspiration, keeping moving down 1-2cm from the RIF to the right costal margin.

Palpate the spleen: use one or both hands starting in the RIF using the edge of the hand, ask the patient to take a deep breath and as they begin, palpate the abdomen. Feel for the spleen edge pass below your hand during inspiration, keeping moving down 1-2cm from the RIF to the left costal margin.

Ballot the kidneys: place your left hand behind the patient's back, and have your right hand over the anterior aspect, pushing your fingers upwards with your left hand and downwards with your right hand.

Palpate the aorta.

Percuss the 9 regions but particularly over the liver, spleen and bladder.

Shifting dullness: this is to check for ascites. Percuss from the umbilicus region to the patients' left flank. If the dullness is noted, this may suggest ascitic fluid. Keep your fingers over the area that became dull and then ask patient to roll on their right side, towards you. You would say you would keep the patient like this for at least 30 seconds and then re-percuss. If there is ascites, the area that was dull will now sound resonant.

Examine the hernia orifices, ask the patient to cough and check if it is reducible.

Auscultation:

Bowel sounds: normal bowel sounds should sound like gurgling; mention you would auscultate for 2 minutes usually. Auscultate near the umbilicus.

Types of bowel sounds:

- Absent: this may be caused by ileus
- Tinkling bowel sounds: due to obstruction

Auscultate for renal bruits over the aorta and renal arteries, above the umbilicus and lateral to the midline on each side.

Mention that you would do special tests if indicated or any suspicion of condition, such as:

- Rovsing's sign: this is the palpation of the LIF which causes pain in the RIF, sign of appendicitis
- Murphy's sign: place fingers at the right costal margin and ask patient to take a deep breath. If the patient suddenly halts their breath due to pain, this may be suggestive of cholecystitis

Legs

Examine the patient's lower legs for signs of pitting oedema (liver cirrhosis, hypoalbuminemia). Check for any erythema nodosum and pyoderma gangrenosum (signs of inflammatory bowel disease)

4 To Complete

- Summarise findings in logical and structured manner
- Offer appropriate diagnosis and differential diagnoses if appropriate
- Further investigations/examinations: full hernia examination, PR examination, external genitalia examination, BOXES, USS
- Thank the patient
- Wash hands

RECTAL (PR) EXAMINATION

1 ICE – Introduction, Consent and Exposure

Introduce yourself: full name and your role

Confirm patient identity (name and date of birth)

Consent for examination

Explain the examination: – 'Today I need to or have been asked to carry out an examination of your back passage. This will involve me inserting a gloved finger into your anus so I can check for any abnormalities. This examination shouldn't be painful. However, it may be slightly uncomfortable. If at any point you would like me to stop, please let me know.'

Appropriate position and exposure: sitting initially, will ask to undress later.

Always have a chaperone present, explain someone else will be in the room due to the nature of the examination.

Check for pain before starting

Wash/gel hands

2 Check Equipment

- Non-sterile gloves
- Paper towel
- Lubricating gel
- Apron

Once everything is ready, ask patient to remove all clothing from waist downwards including underwear and then to cover themselves with a sheet that you will provide (ask them to do this behind the curtains and to call you when they are ready). Once you enter, ask the patient to lie down on their left side with their knees bent up towards their chest. Lift the sheet with their permission.

3 Inspection

Firstly, inspect the perianal area for any skin tags, abscesses, external haemorrhoids, anal fissures, bleeding, fistulas. At this point ask the patient to cough to check for rectal prolapse and internal haemorrhoids.

4 Palpation

Apply gloves and lubricate the examining finger (use the index finger). Before you start, warn the patient that you are about to insert the finger, ask them to take deep breaths. Insert the index finger slowly and gently into the anal canal.

If the patient is male, palpate the prostate gland anteriorly, assess the size, symmetry and consistency of the gland. Normal size is about 2-3cm and should feel like the tip of the nose.

NB enlarged prostate gland can be due to benign prostatic hyperplasia (BPH) or malignancy.

Examine the anal canal, rotate the inserted finger at 360 degrees to assess the entire anal canal. Note/comment on:

- Size
- Location
- Consistency – smooth, hard, irregular
- Lumps– polyps, tumours, internal haemorrhoids, hard impacted stools
- Tenderness

Assess the anal tone: ask the patient to bear down on your finger. You should feel tightness around your finger.

Take the finger out and assess for any bleeding, mucus or stool.

If blood is present, is it dark caused by an upper GI bleeding or bright red caused by a lower GI bleeding such as haemorrhoids or inflammatory bowel disease?

5 To Complete

Provide patient with paper towels and ask them to clean themselves, cover them with the sheet and step out to give them privacy.

Ask them to get dressed and that you will speak once they are done and that the examination is now finished.

Dispose of the equipment and PPE

Wash/gel hands

Thank the patient

Document finding and summarise

Further examination/ investigation: GI examination, colonoscopy, bloods

HERNIA EXAMINATION

1 ICE – Introduction, Consent and Exposure

Introduce yourself: full name and your role

Confirm patient identity (name and date of birth)

Consent for examination

Explain the examination: 'I understand you have noticed a lump on your tummy. I would like to examine this lump and your whole tummy if that's okay. I may also need to examine your groin area (in males) – in this case you will need to remove your underwear at that point.'

Appropriate position and exposure: initially lying flat when examining abdomen and then standing up – explain this to the patient. Remove all clothing from waist upwards.

Always ask about chaperone

Wash/gel hands

2 General Inspection

Patient: comfortable at rest, obvious pain, obvious swelling/lump, scars

Surroundings: TRUS belt – this is a supportive belt used to conservatively manage hernias, medication etc.

3 Examination

Examination of the hernia

Inspection: kneel down to patient's hip level from the side, inspect abdomen and groin for scars from previous surgery, any obvious swellings/lumps – if you notice anything say it out loud and the position, i.e. visible lump on the right side of the lower abdomen. Describe using SPACEPIT.

Palpation: always ask patient about pain before palpating. If there is a lump present, examine that side first. Use the dorsal aspect of your hand and check the temperature on both sides of the abdomen; compare both sides.

For the lump to be a hernia, it must have a cough impulse and has to be reducible. Ask the patient if they can push the lump in. If so, ask them to do this. Then place hand over that area and ask them to cough. If the lump appears you will feel an impulse on the hand and volume increase – cough impulse.

At this point you can tell the examiner that the lump is reducible and has a cough impulse therefore this lump is likely to be a 'hernia'.

Palpate for anatomical landmarks:

- Anterior superior iliac spine (ASIS)
- Pubic symphysis
- Pubic tubercle

To palpate the pubic tubercle, you would have to palpate laterally from pubic symphysis. If a hernia is present, you will have to palpate under it, working inferiorly and laterally.

Comment on the position:

1. Superior medial to pubic tubercle – inguinal hernia
2. Inferior lateral to pubic tubercle – femoral hernia

If it's an inguinal hernia you may need to check whether it is an indirect or direct hernia. At this point reduce the hernia here yourself and press down, and ask the patient to cough. If the hernia reappears then it is a DIRECT hernia, if it doesn't, then it is an INDIRECT hernia.

Auscultate: auscultate bowel sounds over the hernia; do both sides.

You can ask the patient to stand up to observe the hernia in that position.

4 To Complete

Ask them to get dressed and that you will speak once they are done and that the examination is now finished.

Wash/gel hands

Thank the patient

Summarise findings

Further examination/ investigation: GI examination, external genital examination

PREGNANT ABDOMEN

1 ICE – Introduction, Consent and Exposure

Introduce yourself: full name and your role

Confirm patient identity (name and date of birth)

Consent for examination

Explain the examination: 'I would like to examine your tummy today.'

Appropriate position and exposure: expose from xiphisternum to pubic symphysis. The position should be semi recombinant (half lying and sitting). If the patient has hypotensive syndrome, lie them on the left lateral position

Always ask about chaperone

Always check for any pains and how many weeks they are. Gestation?

Wash/gel hands

2 General Inspection

Patient: comfortable at rest, obvious pain, pallor, shortness of breath

3 Abdomen Inspection

Scars, foetal movements, skin changes such as: linea nigra, striae gavidarum, striae albicans – indicate previous pregnancy (silver/whitish in colour) – umbilical inversion caused by the raised intra-abdominal pressure, dilated veins due to increased inferior vena cava.

4 Abdomen Examination

- Fundal height; palpate for the top of the uterus, use the left hand and start at the xiphisternum and work down until the fundus. Measure the fundal height.
- Foetal lie: place your hands on either side. The curved area is the foetal back and lumpy parts are the foetal limbs.
- Presenting part: palpate for this above the pubic symphysis using both hands and apply firm pressure. If it's hard and round it is the head (cephalic), if its soft and broad, it is the buttocks (breech).
- Engagement: if the head is engaged, check with how many fingers out of 5 i.e. 1/5
- Auscultate with a pinard over the anterior shoulder
- Doppler: listen for the heart beat for at least one minute

5 Legs

Check for pitting/peripheral oedema – signs of pre-eclampsia

4 To Complete

Ask them to get dressed and that you will speak once they are done, and that the examination is now finished.

Wash/gel hands

Thank the patient

Summarise findings

Further examination/ investigation: ultrasound scans

BREAST EXAMINATION

1 ICE – Introduction, Consent and Exposure

Introduce yourself: full name and your role

Confirm patient identity (name and date of birth)

Consent for examination

Explain the examination: 'I would like to examine your breasts today, or I understand you have a lump on your breast. Is it okay if I examine you today?'

Appropriate position and exposure: remove clothing from waist upwards including bra. Initial position is sitting and then lying at 30 degrees.

Always ask about chaperone

Always check for any pain

Wash/gel hands

2 General Inspection

Patient: comfortable at rest, weight loss, age

3 Inspection

Do this part while patient is sitting.

Look for asymmetry, local swelling, skin changes such as erythema, dimpling, peau d'orange, scars, nipple changes – inversion, discharge.

Do this with the patient in the following five positions:
- Arms relaxed across lap
- Hands rested on thighs
- Hands actively pressed onto hips (this tenses the pectorals)
- Hands behind the head (this will expose the whole breast and accentuate any dimpling that may be present)
- Ask patient to lift breast, so you can look in the sub-mammary folds

4 Examination

Ask the patient to lie at 30 degrees and ask patient to place the hand under the head on the side that is being examined. Do this for both sides; show them if you have to.

Before starting, check for pain and always start from the normal side.

Examine using both hands, massage into the breast using the flat surface of your hand and use the whole of the 4 fingers.

Move the hands in sections around the breast covering all the quadrants – do this from outside to inside.

Examine the axillary tail using your first two fingers and thumb.

Describe the lump using SPACEPIT.

Ask the patient to try to express any discharge from nipples; check both sides.

5 Lymph Nodes

For this put some gloves on and palpate the nodes with the patient lying flat and then when sitting.

Assess the axillary lymph nodes: ask the patient to hold your right arm while you support the weight of their right arm at their elbow with your right hand. Then place your left arm over your right and place your left hand into their axilla.

Palpate the apical – shoulder joint, lateral – top of arm, medial – centre of axilla, anterior– over breast and posterior lymph node – mid back.

Palpate the supraclavicular lymph node.

6 To Complete

Ask them to get dressed and that you will speak once they are done, and that the examination is now finished.

Wash/gel hands

Thank the patient

Summarise findings

Further examination/ investigation: ultrasound scans/mammogram

Triple assessment: examination, imaging (USS if <35 y/o mammogram if >35 y/o

Tissue sampling (fine needle aspiration if cystic or core biopsy if solid)

MENTAL STATE EXAMINATION

1 ICE – Introduction, Consent and Exposure

Introduce yourself: full name and your role

Confirm patient identity (name and date of birth)

Consent for examination

Wash/gel hands

REMEMBER: A&B, SMT AND PCI

2 A&B – Appearance and Behaviour (You observe this, not ask it)

Observe the following:

- Are they kempt? This is their physical appearance; is there any neglect, usual dress?
- Behaviour: their facial expressions, eye contact, do they seem suspicious, paranoid, irritable, appear to be aggressive?
- Are they distracted, withdrawn or quiet?

3 S SPEECH (Again, you will observe this and not ask this)

- Assess the rate of speech – pressure of speech, is it slow or monotonous or spontaneous?
- Assess the volume, is it too loud or too quiet?
- Is the speech coherent and relevant, do they answer appropriately?
- The flow of speech – any interruptions, shifting topics – 'word salad'?

4 M Mood

You need to ask about their mood and do a depression screen here. (Remember to risk assess their risk to self-harm themselves or others.)

- Subjective: ask how they feel – low or high
- Objective: your opinion from what they are displaying, do they appear low like they say or vice versa? Depressed, elated, euthymic, disinhibition, grandiosity, reactive, flat, blunt affect – when they show one thing but not actually feel that way
- Ask about SAWEMAIL: sleep, appetite, weight loss, energy, mood, anhedonia, irritability, libido
- Assess SADPERSONS

Factor	Points
Sex – male	1
Age <19 or > 45	1
Depression or hopelessness	2
Previous suicide attempt	1
Excessive alcohol or drug abuse	1
Rational thinking los	2
Separated, divorced or widowed	1
Organised or serious attempt	2
No social support	1
Stated future intent	2

Score 6-8: full emergency psychiatric evaluation/treatment
Score of 9 or more: immediate psychiatric hospitalisation

5 T Thoughts

Don't go straight into this, start like this: 'Sometimes when we feel low, we can hear and see things that are not there and also do things that are out of character, so I will need to ask about…'

- Check for delusions: Have you noticed having any strange thoughts, or thoughts that others may find strange? Can anyone interfere with or hear your thoughts? Do you feel you are in control of your actions? Do you ever get thoughts that you keep thinking about over and over? Are there any actions that you need to do repeatedly?
- Form: coherence, muddled, flight of ideas, preoccupied with thoughts-,any disordered thoughts?
- Content: suicidal thoughts or deliberate self-harm (DSH) or towards others, delusions, insertion/withdrawal. 'When watching TV, do you feel like they are talking to you?'
- Obsessions: acceptable ideas, pursued by patient beyond bounds of reason and causes suffering/disturbed functioning – preoccupations/ruminations

6 P Perceptions

Check for hallucinations: 'Have you ever heard or seen anything you cannot explain?' 'Do you hear people talk that are not in the room?' 'Do you feel that any specific event may have a direct message for you?'

- Perceptions: in their own head
- Hallucinations/illusions: auditory, visual, tactile, olfactory, gustatory or absence of external stimuli
- Pseudo hallucination
- Hypnagogic: waking up hearing your name
- Hypnopompic: waking up hearing something and it's not there

7 C Cognition

You can do a quick MMSE here or 6 CIT

Check:

- Concentration and attention/orientation
- Confusion
- Memory

8 I Insight

- Are they aware of their illness and that they are unwell? What do they think is going on?
- Do they understand the need for their treatment/medications?
- Are they willing for treatment?

9 To Complete

- Summarise findings
- Thank patient
- Wash/gel hands
- Further investigations: bloods etc. to exclude any organic causes of the current mental problems (Bloods – FBC, U&Es, LFTS, blood glucose, TFTS, Vitamin B12, folate, iron studies, syphilis) CT/MRI

6 CIT Cognitive Impairment Test

1. What year is it?
2. What month is it?
3. Give patient an address and ask them to remember till the end – John Smith, 42 High St, Bedford
4. What time is it? (within the hour)
5. Count backwards from 201-1

Say the months of the year in reverse

1. Repeat address given earlier

Score out of 28
0– 7 normal, 8 or more – significant

Mini Mental State Exam – MMSE

1. Orientation
2. Registration
3. Attention
4. Recall
5. Language
6. Copying

VERIFICATION OF DEATH

1. Identify patient from and confirm with wrist band
2. Check that the patient's eyes are closed and that there are no signs of life
3. Make note – no respiratory effort
4. No response to verbal stimuli
5. No response to pain stimuli
6. No palpable carotid pulse
7. Dilated and fixed pupils bilaterally
8. No heart sounds heard during 2 minutes of auscultation
9. No breathing sounds noted during 3 minutes of auscultation
10. Document death time and date

3

Procedural Skills

URINE DIPSTICK

1 ICE – Introduction, Consent and Exposure

Introduce yourself: full name and your role

Confirm patient identity (name and date of birth)

Consent for examination

Explain procedure: They will most likely hand you the urine sample. 'I understand you have a urine sample for me, I would like to dip that using special equipment to check for any abnormalities such as infection.'

Wash/gel hands

Wear gloves

2 Inspect the urine

Observe the:

- Colour – dark, pale, any blood, pus, sedimentation, cloudy
- Smell to check for any foul odour – sweet smell – ketonuria

3 Dipstick

- Check the expiry on the dipstick container and take one out
- Dip the dipstick into the urine and ensure all the squares are covered by the urine
- Remove the dipstick and place horizontally on a tissue
- Allow at least 1-2 minutes and read the results against the dipstick container
- Document results and discard all waste into the waste bin
- Take gloves off and wash hands
- Thank the patient and if the station states to explain results then do so

4 Explanation

- Summarise findings
- If there are signs of infection, explain that to the patient and the next step in terms of management of further investigations

INTRAMUSCULAR INJECTION

1 ICE – Introduction, Consent and Exposure

Introduce yourself: full name and your role

Confirm patient identity (name and date of birth)

Consent for examination

Explain procedure: 'Today I need to give you an injection that will go in the top of your arm, you will feel a sharp scratch.'

Wash/gel hands

Allergy check always when administering drugs

Check for any bleeding disorders or on any blood thinners

Check for any contraindications for IMs

Check which side is preferred – left or right?

Exposure: the deltoid part of the preferred arm if deltoid

Position: sitting

2 Preparation of the Tray

Wash hands

Clean the tray

Gather all the equipment you require:

- The drug (check expiry date, batch number, allergies and prescription)
- Non-sterile gloves
- Apron
- Syringe
- Needles – green to draw up, blue to inject
- Alcohol wipe
- Gauze or cotton wool
- Sharps bin

3 Final Checks

Remember the Rs

1. Right person – confirm patient details, check against wrist band or system. Use at least 2 identifiers
2. Right drug – check labelled drug against the prescription and the expiry date
3. Right dose – check the dose against the prescription
4. Right time – check if it's the correct time and check if they have had previous dose and when
5. Right route – check the route is appropriate for the type of medication that is being administered
6. Right to refuse – make sure you gain valid consent
7. Right documentation

4 Performing the IM injection

- Wash hands, put on gloves and aprons
- Draw the medication up using the drawing needle
- Remove the drawing needle and dispose in sharps bin – (NEVER RE-SHEATH) then attach the injecting needle
- Choose site i.e. deltoid, ventrogluteal (not used much), vastus lateralis
- Clean site with the alcohol wipe for 30 seconds and let air dry (this can vary on hospital policies as WHO doesn't recommend it, but for OSCEs do it!)
- Apply traction on skin, z-track, so pull skin using dominant hand away from the injection site, to separate skin layers – so medication can be administered into muscle layer. If patient is elderly or reduced muscle mass, bunch the skin instead.
- Hold the injection like a dart in your dominant hand, and inject at 90-degree angle. Insert the injection firmly and quickly, but WARN THE PATIENT with 'sharp scratch', ensure the bevel is facing upwards, leave one third of the shaft exposed (this may vary patient to patient.)
- Aspirate to ensure that you have not hit a blood vessel. If there is blood, you need to discard and restart.
- If there is not blood, proceed, inject medication slowly over 10 seconds
- Remove the needle and dispose into a sharps bin
- Release the traction and apply gentle pressure with cotton wool over the injection site
- DO NOT RUB
- If they are on any blood thinners – apply pressure for 2–3 minutes (mention this)
- Dispose of all equipment appropriately

5 To Complete

Explain it is finished

Thank patient

Remove PPE and wash/gel hands

Explain to the patient about possible reactions which can be normal and last up to 48 hours, such as haematoma formation, local irritation, systemic symptoms such as cold–flu like symptoms, local pain and rarely anaphylaxis. Advise them to seek urgent medical care if they notice lip or tongue swelling or any breathing difficulties. Also, if the common symptoms persist, inform that they should seek medical advice for this.

Document details

SUBCUTANEOUS INJECTION

1 ICE – Introduction, Consent and Exposure

Introduce yourself: full name and your role

Confirm patient identity (name and date of birth)

Consent for examination

Explain procedure: 'Today I need to give you an injection that will go in your tummy/upper thighs, you will feel a sharp scratch.'

Wash/gel hands

Allergy check always when administrating drugs

Check for any bleeding disorders or on any blood thinners

Check for any contraindications for SCs

Check which side is preferred – left or right?

Exposure: correct exposure of site

Position: sitting

2 Preparation of the Tray

Wash hands

Clean the tray

Gather all the equipment you require:

- The drug (check expiry date, batch number, allergies and prescription)
- Non-sterile gloves
- Apron
- Usually, a pre-filled syringe, if not then also the following
- Syringe
- Needles – one to draw up and one for injecting
- Alcohol wipe
- Sharps bin

3 Final Checks

Remember the Rs

- Right person – confirm patient details, check against wrist band or system. Use at least 2 identifiers
- Right drug – check labelled drug against the prescription and the expiry date
- Right dose – check the dose against the prescription
- Right time – check if it's the correct time and check if they have had previous dose and when
- Right route – check the route is appropriate for the type of medication that is being administered
- Right to refuse – make sure you gain valid consent
- Right documentation

4 Performing the SC injection

- Wash hands, put on gloves and aprons
- Draw the medication up using the drawing needle
- Remove the drawing needle and dispose in sharps bin – (NEVER RE-SHEATH) then attach the injecting needle
- Choose site i.e. abdomen, upper outer aspect of arm, upper outer aspect of thigh
- Clean site with the alcohol wipe
- Pinch the skin using your thumb and index finger using your non dominant hand. This is to lift the subcutaneous layer.
- Hold the injection at 45 to 90 degrees angle in your dominant hand and insert the injection firmly and quickly, but WARN THE PATIENT with 'sharp scratch', ensure the bevel is facing upwards, leave one third of the shaft exposed (this may vary patient to patient)
- Remove the needle and dispose into a sharps bin
- Release the traction and apply gentle pressure with cotton wool over the injection site

- DO NOT RUB
- If they are on any blood thinners – apply pressure for 2-3 minutes (mention this)
- Dispose of all equipment appropriately

5 To Complete

Explain it is finished

Thank patient

Remove PPE and wash/gel hands

Explain to the patient about possible reactions which can be normal and last up to 48 hours, such as haematoma formation, local irritation, local pain and rarely anaphylaxis. Advise them to seek urgent medical care if they notice lip or tongue swelling or any breathing difficulties. Also, if the common symptoms persist, inform them that they should seek medical advice for this.

Document details

VENEPUNCTURE

(NB in this station they may have an anxious patient. Although you want to carry out this procedure in a safe, systematic and aseptic manner, remember you need to communicate. This may be a procedural OSCE station but at the same time they will be assessing your communication skills. If the patient is anxious, acknowledge that, reassure them, ask if they want a nurse in here with you for support.)

1 ICE – Introduction, Consent and Exposure

Introduce yourself: full name and your role

Confirm patient identity (name and date of birth)

Consent for examination

Explain procedure: 'Today I need to take some bloods from your arm, is that okay?'

Check allergies

Check for any bleeding disorders or if on any blood thinners

Check which arm they prefer to be used

Exposure: correct exposure of site

Position: sitting

2 Preparation

Wash and gel hands

Position the patient's arm in an extended position

Inspect the site i.e. the antecubital fossa (ACF), always start proximally for bloods

Apply the tourniquet 4–5cm above the area for venepuncture

Palpate for an appropriate vein – ensure it is soft and bouncy

Release the tourniquet

Wash hands and apply gloves

Clean the chosen site with an alcohol wipe for 30 seconds and allow to air dry for 30 seconds

Clean the whole area

After this point, ensure not to touch this cleaned site

3 Blood Taking

Attach the needle to the vacutainer

Re-apply tourniquet

Unsheathe needle and anchor the vein from above, below or on the side by gently pulling using non dominant hand

Before inserting the needle, WARN THE PATIENT with 'sharp scratch'

Insert the needle at a 20–30 degree angle with the bevel facing upwards

Advance the needle 1–2 mm. Once the flashback is observed, lower the needle and anchor the needle to the patient's skin

Attach your blood bottles (remember the order Blue, Yellow, Purple, Red)

Once all bottles have been taken, release the tourniquet

Withdraw the needle and apply pressure over site with a swab

Ask patient to apply firm pressure, while you dispose of sharps in the sharps bin

If the patient is on blood thinners, apply pressure for 2–3 minutes

Remove the swab/cotton wool, and use a new one – apply tape over it or apply a plaster over the venepuncture site

Discard all other waste into the appropriate bins

4 To Complete

Thank the patient

Wash and gel hands

Label bottles

If it's a failed attempt, state that you will take two attempts and after that you ask another clinician or health care professional to have a go.

12 LEAD ECG PROCEDURE

1 ICE – Introduction, Consent and Exposure

Introduce yourself: full name and your role

Confirm patient identity (name and date of birth)

Consent for examination

Explain procedure: 'Today I would like to take a tracing of your heart, which will involve applying some sticky tabs to your chest, wrists and ankle. It will not harm you in any way.' (If they are male and have hair on their chest, warn them that you may need to shave small areas in order to apply the sticky tabs.) Always ask if they have any questions.

Check for any current chest pains and acknowledge their pain and tell them you will have some pain relief sorted afterwards.

Exposure: behind the curtains, ask them to take everything off from waist upwards, including bra

Position: lying at a 45-degree angle

Wash and gel hands

2 Placement of Electrodes

Although it's a 12-lead ECG, only 10 electrodes are used: 4 on the 4 limbs and 6 chest leads.

Before starting check all the sticky tabs are in date and ensure patient's skin is clean and free from any dirt. Shave if needed.

You must palpate all anatomical locations for the electrodes for OSCE purposes so the examiner can see that you know the exact locations.

Limbs leads:

RIDE YOUR GREEN BIKE

- Right wrist – RED electrode
- Left wrist – YELLOW electrode
- Left ankle – GREEN electrode
- Right ankle – BLACK electrode

Chest leads:

- V1 – count from Angle of Louis (2nd intercostal space – ICS), 4th ICS at the right sternal border
- V2 – 4th ICS at the left sternal border
- V3 – in between V2 and V4
- V4 – place V4 before V3, 5th ICS in the mid clavicular line
- V5 – 5th ICS, anterior to axillary line – same horizontal plane as V4 and V5
- V6 – 5th ICS, midaxillary line – same horizontal plane as V4 and V5

To prevent the electrodes from being pulled off, be sure to connect the wires to the electrodes in an organised manner, i.e. all chest electrodes should be placed with the wires facing downwards and limb leads facing upwards.

3 Recording

Check all wires are attached against the screen/monitor for ECG machine

Check patient details are logged in and say you would check that there is paper in the printer and the standard is correct

Ask patient to lie still and relax with arms down by their sides

Press record

4 To Complete

Tell the patient you are finished and ask if you should take the tabs off, or will they?

Hand them some tissue to wipe the gel off

Ask them to get changed and thank them

On the recording check patient details – name, DOB, patient ID, gender, not any pain or severity of pain.

Wash and gel hands

5 Interpret ECG

If you are asked to interpret an ECG:

Do it systematically

- Check patient details – name, DOB, gender, time and date
- Rate
- Rhythm
- Axis – normal or left or right axis deviation
- Present P wave
- PR interval
- QRS complex
- P and QRS wave corresponding with one another
- Q wave and ST segments
- T wave – any inversions
- Summarise findings and suggestion of possible diagnosis

PEAK FLOW

1 ICE – Introduction, Consent and Exposure

Introduce yourself: full name and your role

Confirm patient identity (name and date of birth)

Gain consent to proceed and check understanding

Explain procedure: 'Today I would like to assess how well your lungs work using a very simple piece of equipment.'

Check for any recent chest infections, any recent use of steroids or bronchodilators

Position: Sitting in a chair

Wash and gel hands

2 The Procedure

Explain everything first and then hand them the meter

Set the peak flow meter to zero

Ensure you have a clean and unused mouth piece

Ask the patient to stand upright during the peak flow test

Ask the patient to take a deep breath in and out to begin with

Then ask them to take a deep breath in and form a tight seal around the mouth piece with their lips

Ensure they hold the meter horizontally without blocking the dial with their fingers

Then ask them to breathe out fast and as hard as they can for 10 seconds

Ask them to do this at least 3 times, each time reset the meter in between

Hand the meter to patient so they can do all above

3 To Complete

To document on the nomogram, you will need to ask the patient about their height, age, weight and gender

Ask the patient to keep a diary of their daily readings, twice a day

Check patient understands how to use the peak flow

Thank patient

Wash/gel hands

ARTERIAL BLOOD GAS

1 ICE – Introduction, Consent and Exposure

Introduce yourself: full name and your role

Confirm patient identity (name and date of birth)

Gain consent to proceed

Explain procedure: 'Today I would like to do a special blood test, which will involve me taking bloods from one of your arteries which is located in your wrist. It may be slighter more painful than a normal blood test.'

Ask which is their non-dominant hand

Check for any allergies, check for any bleeding disorders and if they are on any blood thinning medications

Position: Sitting in a chair/lying

Wash and gel hands

2 The Procedure

Gather your equipment, firstly clean the tray

Equipment: gloves, apron, alcohol wipe, a heparinised syringe with a needle, rubber bung, syringe cap, tape, cotton wool

Before starting: state you would like to do the Modified Allen's test

Modified Allen's test: This test is used to check the patency and flow of the artery in the hands

- Test one hand at a time
- Elevate the hand and ask the patient to clench their first for 30 seconds
- Apply pressure over both the radial and ulnar artery simultaneously, so that you are occluding both arteries
- While the hand is elevated, ask patient to open their fist and the hand should appear blanched
- Release the ulnar pressure while radial pressure is still maintained; the colour should return to the hands within 5 to 15 seconds
- If colour returns within time frame, this is a normal Allen's test

Position patient's arm resting on a pillow, with their arm extended

Palpate the radial artery

Clean the site for 30 seconds

Put on gloves and apron

Always mention you can also administer lidocaine before doing the ABG

Attach the ABG syringe to the needle, expel the heparin to prep the needle

Re-palpate the radial artery with your non dominant hand

Hold the ABG syringe like a pencil, angle at 45 degrees

WARN THE PATIENT with 'sharp scratch'

TIP: if using 3 fingers to palpate radial artery, if you lift your middle finger that's usually a good spot to insert needle

Once inserted, the syringe should begin to self-fill

Once sufficient amount is collected, remove the needle and apply firm pressure over site using a gauze for 3–5 minutes

Safety guard needle and remove needle from syringe, discard into the sharps bin

Place the cap over the syringe head and label the sample

3 To Complete

Examiner may present you with some ABG results, so ensure to know the normal and possible abnormal readings from an ABG and what they can mean

Remove PPE, wash/gel hands

Thank patient

Ensure to reassure patient throughout, especially if they appear to be anxious. Remember communication, even during an examination station, is KEY.

FEMALE CATHETERISATION

1 ICE – Introduction, Consent and Exposure

Introduce yourself: full name and your role

Confirm patient identity (name and date of birth)

Gain consent to proceed

Tell them there will be a chaperone present

Explain procedure: start with checking patient's knowledge already, 'Has anyone explained what will happen today? I would like to insert a catheter into your bladder. It's a thin and flexible tube, I will be using some local anaesthetic gel to make it less uncomfortable. The tube will be attached to a bag, so that we can monitor your urine outflow. The procedure may be slightly uncomfortable but shouldn't be painful. If you want me to stop at any point, please let me know and I will stop.'

Check for any allergies, particularly latex gloves. And check if patient is in any current pain.

Position: lying position

Wash and gel hands

Indications:
- Collection of sterile urine sample
- Urinary tract obstruction
- Bladder decompression
- Urinary retention
- Urinary incompetence i.e. due to spinal cord injury
- Monitor urinary output – post surgery, sepsis, critically ill patients

Equipment:

- Procedure trolley – clean with alcohol wipe
- Plastic tray – clean with alcohol wipe
- Disposable plastic apron
- Two pairs of sterile gloves
- Protective waterproof sheet
- At least 10ml 0.9% sodium chloride (saline) solution for injection
- 10ml sterile water, drawn into a syringe
- 1% sterile lidocaine anaesthetic lubricating gel, drawn into a syringe
- Urinary catheter (of appropriate type, size and length)
- Sterile catheter pack (containing cotton wool balls, gallipot (small pot), sterile gauze swabs, sterile fenestrated drapes, urine bowl)
- Sterile closed urinary drainage system (e.g. catheter bag)
- Urine collection bowl

2 Equipment Preparation

Check the expiry dates on the catheter, sterile water, saline and lubricating gel

Wash your hands

Put apron on

Open catheter pack on top of the clean trolley, only touch the outer packaging

Ensure to use aseptic non-touch technique throughout

Empty the catheter and syringes, lidocaine gel and sterile water into the sterile field

Keep the catheter packet, which will be needed for documentation on the patient's notes later

3 Patient Preparation

Ask the patient to remove clothing from waist below including underwear. Ask them to do this behind the curtains and then cover themselves with a sheet provided. Ensure the curtains are closed. Ask the patient to let you know when they are ready.

When you enter, ask the patient to lie back, put their feet together and bring their heels towards their bottom and then part their knees (Lithotomy position).

Place a urine collection bowl on the bed below the patient's genitalia, in between their legs.

KEY: maintain patient dignity throughout and minimise exposure when you can

Ask your chaperone now to remove the sheet, so you can maintain sterility

REMEMBER THE 7 Cs

1. Confirm – name and DOB
2. Consent
3. Check understanding
4. Chaperone
5. Behind the curtains
6. Lie down on couch
7. Cover patient

4 Procedure

Wash or gel your hands and put sterile gloves on

Place your cotton wools into the gallipot from the pack

Pour over the 0.9% saline solution

Expose the patient's genitalia and using your non dominant hand part the labia

Insert the syringe nozzle of lubricating gel into the urethral meatus using your dominant hand and slowly disperse the syringe content into the urethra

Dispose of your gloves and apply a new pair of sterile gloves

Tear the plastic covering of the catheter wrapping carefully and only expose the tip. Position the distal end of catheter into the urine collection bowl

Now warn the patient that you will be inserting the catheter and again part the labia using your non dominant hand and insert the catheter tip into the urethral meatus

Slowly advance the catheter until it reaches bladder and you see a urine flow

Think of your hands as clean (dominant hand) and unclean hand (non-dominant hand)

Secure the catheter inside the bladder by inflating the balloon.

Connect the 10ml syringe which contains sterile water to the balloon port and gently inflate the catheter balloon

During this observe the patient closely and ask them to let you know of any pain, as this may suggest incorrect position

Attach the catheter to the catheter bag. Position the bag below the level of the bladder to ensure drainage of urine. Secure the bag on a catheter stand.

5 To Complete

Clean surrounding area and pass some tissue to patient to clean themselves

Check that the patient is comfortable and the surrounding area is clean

Discard any waste in appropriate waste bins

Thank patient and ask them to flag up any pain or leakage

Remove your gloves and wash hands

Document the procedure in patient's notes, ensure to document the date, time, indication, catheter size, local anaesthetic details, amount of urine and the appearance, any issues or complications and a planned removal date. Document patient consent and name of chaperone.

MALE CATHETERISATION

1 ICE – Introduction, Consent and Exposure

Introduce yourself: full name and your role

Confirm patient identity (Name and date of birth)

Gain consent to proceed

Tell them there will be a chaperone present

Explain procedure: start with checking patient's knowledge already, 'Has anyone explained what will happen today? I would like to insert a catheter into your bladder, it's a thin and flexible tube, I will be using some local anaesthetic gel to make it less uncomfortable. The tube will be attached to a bag, so that we can monitor your urine outflow. The procedure may be slightly uncomfortable but shouldn't be painful. If you want me to stop at any point, please let me know and I will stop.'

Check for any allergies, particularly latex gloves. And check if patient is in any current pain.

Position: lying position

Wash and gel hands

Indications
- Collection of sterile urine sample
- Urinary tract obstruction

- Bladder decompression
- Urinary retention
- Urinary incompetence i.e. due to spinal cord injury
- Monitor urinary output – post surgery, sepsis, critically ill patients

Equipment

- Procedure trolley – clean with alcohol wipe
- Plastic tray – clean with alcohol wipe
- Disposable plastic apron
- Two pairs of sterile gloves
- Protective waterproof sheet
- At least 10ml 0.9% sodium chloride (saline) solution for injection
- 10ml sterile water, drawn into a syringe
- 1% sterile lidocaine anaesthetic lubricating gel, drawn into a syringe
- Urinary catheter (of appropriate type, size and length)
- Sterile catheter pack (containing cotton wool balls, gallipot (small pot), sterile gauze swabs, sterile fenestrated drapes, urine bowl)
- Sterile closed urinary drainage system (e.g. catheter bag)
- Urine collection bowl

2 Equipment Preparation

Check the expiry dates on the catheter, sterile water, saline and lubricating gel

Wash your hands

Put on apron

Open catheter pack on top of the clean trolley, only touch the outer packaging

Ensure to use aseptic non-touch technique throughout

Empty the catheter and syringes, lidocaine gel and sterile water into the sterile field

Keep the catheter packet, which will be needed for documentation on the patient's notes later

3 Patient Preparation

Ask the patient to remove clothing from waist below including underwear. Ask them to do this behind the curtains and then cover themselves with a sheet provided. Ensure the curtains are closed. Ask the patient to let you know when they are ready.

When you enter, ask the patient to lie back, and extend their legs and slightly apart.

Do not uncover patient at this point

Place a protective waterproof sheet under the patient's buttocks

KEY: maintain patient dignity throughout and minimise exposure when you can

Ask your chaperone now to remove the sheet, so you can maintain sterility

REMEMBER THE 7 Cs

1. Confirm – name and DOB
2. Consent
3. Check understanding
4. Chaperone
5. Behind the curtains
6. Lie down on couch
7. Cover patient

4 Procedure

Wash or gel your hands and put sterile gloves on

Place your cotton wools into the gallipot from the pack

Pour over the 0.9% saline solution

Expose the patient's genitalia and using your non dominant hand retract the foreskin if there is one and use a sterile swab to hold the penis in place

With your dominant hand, pick up a cotton wool ball. With a single stroke, clean part of the glans ensuring that you clean away from the urethral meatus. Repeat the process with fresh cotton until you are satisfied the glans has been cleaned.

Open the sterile drape and place the hole in the drape over the penis so it is surrounded. Dispose of the cotton wool balls in clinical waste. Position a sterile urine collection bowl below the penis, on top of the drape and between the patient's legs.

Use a fresh sterile gauze swab in your non dominant hand and hold penis vertically. Insert the syringe nozzle of lubricating gel into the urethral meatus using your dominant hand and slowly disperse the syringe contents into the urethra.

Continue to hold the penis in place, so the gel doesn't leak from the penis. Allow 3–4 minutes for the anaesthetic to set (mention this to examiner) and then let go of the penis

Dispose of your gloves and apply a new pair of sterile gloves

Tear the plastic covering of the catheter wrapping carefully and only expose the tip. Position the distal end of catheter into the urine collection bowl

Now warn the patient that you will be inserting the catheter, again holding penis vertically with your non dominant hand using the gauze. Using your dominant hand insert the catheter tip into the urethral meatus

Slowly advance the catheter until it reaches bladder and you see a urine flow. In males this usually occurs once it reaches the catheter bifurcation point.

(RETRACT WRAPPER AS YOU GO ALONG)

Think of your hands as clean (dominant hand) and unclean hand (non-dominant hand)

Secure the catheter inside the bladder by inflating the balloon

Connect the 10ml syringe which contains sterile water to the balloon port and gently inflate the catheter balloon.

During this observe the patient closely and ask them to let you know of any pain, as this may suggest incorrect position

Attach the catheter to the catheter bag. Position the bag below the level of the bladder to ensure drainage of urine. Secure the bag on a catheter stand.

5 To Complete

Clean surrounding area and pass some tissue to patient to clean themselves

Check that the patient is comfortable and the surrounding area is clean

Discard any waste in appropriate waste bins

Thank patient and ask them to flag up any pain or leakage

Remove your gloves and wash hands

Document the procedure in patient's notes, ensure to document the date, time, indication, catheter size, local anaesthetic details, amount of urine and the appearance, any issues or complications and a planned removal date. Document patient consent and name of chaperone.

CANNULATION

1 ICE – Introduction, Consent and Exposure

Introduce yourself: full name and your role

Confirm patient identity (name and date of birth)

Check for any allergies, particularly latex gloves, and check if patient is in any current pain.

Gain consent to proceed

Explain procedure: 'I would like to put a needle into the back of your hand. This will allow me to put a little plastic tube in your vein so we can deliver medication to you quickly and efficiently.'

Position: sitting or lying position

Ask about chaperone

Wash and gel hands

2 Preparation

Wear gloves and apron

Open the dressing pack and place the cannula, dressing and other required items into a clean tray

Ensure to clean tray before starting (will lose marks if you don't)

Prepare the normal saline flush using a drawing up syringe that is provided

If there is an extension set, attach this to the flush and prime the extension line

Now place a pillow if available under the patient's arm and check they are comfortable

Place a sheet under the arm to keep area clean from any possible spillages

3 Find the Vein

You must ensure the vein you want to use is suitable – bouncy – and the area is clean, no skin execrations or wound over the site

You can ask if they have a preference of which side, although it may not always be possible to adhere to due to not knowing which side will have better veins

Always start distally for cannula, i.e. back of the hand

Inspect for a suitable vein and apply tourniquet above the site and palpate for a vein

Once you have identified a suitable vein, release the tourniquet and clean the site for 30 seconds using an alcohol wipe, and allow the site to air dry while you prepare for cannulation. Clean from the centre of the site, moving outwards, covering a suitable surface area. Ensure NOT to re palpate or touch the cleaned site after this.

4 Cannulation

Remove gloves and wash hands again

Apply fresh non-sterile gloves and apron (mention to the examiner you would change your apron at this point too)

Re apply tourniquet (remember a tourniquet should never stay on for longer than 2 minutes, hence the reason you take it off in between, as it can take longer than 2 minutes sometimes)

Remove the sheath from the cannula

Open the cannula, slightly withdraw needle. Unscrew the cap at the back of the cannula and place upright in the tray

Anchor the vein using your non-dominant hand from below; do this by gently pulling the skin distal to the insertion site

Before you proceed, WARN THE PATIENT with 'sharp scratch'

Insert the cannula directly above the vein, pierce the skin at an angle of 15–30 degrees, bevel facing upwards. Observe for the first flashback in the cannula chamber.

Lower the angle of the cannula and advance the needle further 2mm after observing first flashback

Then withdraw the needle partially, but make sure the needle end is still withing the plastic tube of the cannula

Now advance the cannula into the vein fully

Release the tourniquet and place some gauze under the cannula

Apply direct pressure over the vein to prevent any bleeding from the cannula tip

Gently pull the introducer needle backwards while holding the cannula wing in position

Dispose of the introducer needle into a sharps bin

Apply the adhesive stickers that are found on the dressing and secure the cannula wings in a vertical manner, so that you do not block the insertion site

The site needs to be visible, so we can continually check for any phlebitis or issues over the site

5 Flush the Cannula

Inject the saline into the cannula using the flush that you prepared earlier. Check that the patient has no pain or discomfort when doing this. Also check for any leaking from the cannula, as this may suggest extravasation

If all is well, apply the dressing, use sticky tab to put date on and attach to dressing

6 To Complete

Tidy up station and dispose of any waste in appropriate bins

Remove any PPE

Hand/gel hands

Thank patient

Keep cannula pack for documentation and say you will now document the procedure in the patient's notes.

SUTURING

1 ICE – Introduction, Consent and Exposure

Introduce yourself: full name and your role

Confirm patient identity (name and date of birth)

Check for any allergies, particularly latex gloves and any issues with local anaesthetic. And check if patient is in any current pain, acknowledge this and say you will organise some help/pain relief for this.

May need to check tetanus status

Gain consent to proceed

Explain procedure: 'I need to put some stitches in to close your wound. It may be slightly uncomfortable but before we start, we will give you an injection to numb the area.'

Position: sitting or lying position

Ask about chaperone

Wash and gel hands

2 Procedure

Prepare a sterile field

Put on apron and gloves

Check that the site/wound is clean, any signs of infection

Local anaesthetic (to be prescribed by a prescriber) check the expiry date, dose, ml

Draw up the anaesthetic and inject the anaesthetic – ensure to cover sufficiently and check sensation after injection (the examiner will most likely ask you to leave this part)

Start the sutures once patient confirms site is numb – ensure to use correct technique. Many good YouTube videos available.

Ensure the sutures are evenly spaced and there are equal bites either side of the wound

The sutures must be secure and perpendicular across the entire wound

Any excess suture length should be trimmed and close the wound appropriately

3 Post Procedure

Dispose of all sharps in sharps bin

Provide patient with appropriate wound care tetanus status, keeping the site clean and dry

Inform them of how many sutures were put in and that they will be removed in 5–7 days, unless they are self-dissolving sutures.

Safety net – explain signs of infection. If the wound was to split or open they should seek urgent medical attention

4 To Complete

Thank patient

Remove PPE and dispose of correctly

Document the procedure into patient's notes and include: the site, location, number of sutures, dose of local anaesthetic used, removal date and review date

SPECULUM EXAMINATION

1 ICE – Introduction, Consent and Exposure

Introduce yourself: full name and your role

Confirm patient identity (name and date of birth)

Check for any allergies, particularly latex gloves and lubricating gel

Explain procedure: 'Today I will need to do a speculum examination. This will involve me inserting a small, lubricated piece of plastic equipment into the vagina, so that I can observe the neck of the womb and look for any changes or abnormalities. This procedure should not be painful; however, it may be slightly uncomfortable. If you would like me to stop at any point, please let me know. Post-procedure there may be slight vaginal bleeding which is absolutely normal. A chaperone will be present throughout.'

Gain consent to proceed

Check if they have any questions

Ask if they are in any pain, any possible chance of pregnancy

Before starting ask patient to empty their bladder if they have not already done so

Position: lithotomy position

Exposure: explain to them that you will require all clothing from waist below to be removed including their underwear. They will change behind the curtains and lie on the couch, covering themselves with a sheet provided

Wash and gel hands

2 Equipment Needed

- Non-sterile gloves
- Apron
- Lubricant
- Speculum – there are different sizes
- Light source
- Paper towel

Ask patient to get ready and to let you know when they are, and always check before opening curtains

3 Vulval Inspection

Once patient is in the correct lithotomy position: 'Bring your heels towards your bottom and let your knees fall to the sides'

Put on pair of non-sterile gloves

Inspect the vulva for abnormalities: ulcers, abnormal vaginal discharge, scarring, vaginal atrophy, white lesions, masses, Bartholin's cyst, rashes, Lichen sclerosus

Observe for vaginal prolapse: ask the patient to cough and observe for a bulge that may protrude the vagina

4 Inserting Speculum

Before starting warn the patient that you will insert the speculum, and ask again at this point if this is okay

Use your left hand – index finger and thumb to separate the labia

Gently insert the speculum sideways, ensure that the blades are closed and angled downwards

Once inserted, rotate the speculum back to 90 degrees, so that the handle is facing upwards

Open the speculum blades until the cervix can be seen clearly

Tighten the speculum by locking the nut, so that the position of the blades is fixed

5 Cervix Visualisation

Identify the cervical os – if it is open this may indicate an incomplete or inevitable miscarriage

Inspect for any erosions around the os – ectropion

Cervical masses

Ulcers

And abnormal discharge

6 Removal of Speculum

Loosen the lock and partially close the blades

Rotate the speculum to 90 degrees

Gently remove the speculum, let the patient know you are removing the speculum. As you are doing this inspect the vaginal walls

Cover the patient with a sheet and explain that the procedure is now finished, leave them to get dressed. Provide paper towels so they can clean themselves

Dispose of all waste appropriately

7 To Complete

Thank patient

Dispose of PPE

Wash/gel hands

Document into patient notes – mention you will do this

Summarise your findings

Further investigations: urinalysis, swabs, smear test, USS

NASOGASTRIC TUBE

1 ICE – Introduction, Consent and Exposure

Introduce yourself: full name and your role

Confirm patient identity (name and date of birth)

Check for any allergies, particularly latex gloves and lubricating gel

Explain procedure: today I will need to put a nasogastric tube in. This will involve me putting a small tube through the nose, which will go down your throat into your stomach, (explain the reason why, i.e. the indication) and explain it shouldn't be painful but may be slightly uncomfortable. If at any point they would like you to stop, to raise their hand and you will stop.

Tell them you will ask them to swallow repeatedly

Inform them of risks and check for contraindications

Risks: sores around the nose due to tape etc, and tube may hit the lungs

Contraindications: varicies, base of skull fracture and recent epistaxis

Gain consent to proceed

Check if they have any questions

Ask if they are in any pain before starting

Position: sitting upright

Wash and gel hands

2 Preparation

Wash and gel hands

Clean the tray inside and outside

Gather all the relevant equipment:

- Apron and gloves
- Vomit bowl
- Cup of water with a straw
- Nasogastric tube
- Lubricant
- 10ml syringe – for aspiration
- Saline filled with 10ml to flush
- pH paper strip to check position
- Tape – to tape down tube

Wash hands and open all the packaging and place equipment in the tray

3 Patient Preparation and Procedure

Sit patient up – straight and upright

Ask the patient to blow their nose and provide a tissue

Measure for the tube size using the tube – from the patient's tip of the nose to the ear lobe to the xiphisternum (remember the measurement)

Wash hands

Put on gloves

Lubricate the tube with gel

Ask the patient to hold the cup of water and place straw in their mouth

Warn the patient that you are starting

Gently push tube into the nostrils as close to horizontally as possible

The patient will start to gag when the tube reaches the back of their throat

Ask them to keep taking sips via the straw and keep on swallowing

Push the tube down faster when swallowing

Throughout ensure to communicate and reassure patient

Continue advancing tube until it reaches the measured measurement

Confirm the correct tube placement – in the stomach and not the lungs – by using these methods:
- pH paper – aspirate gastric contents and drop onto pH paper, the pH must be under 6. If aspiration fails, ask the patient to lie on their left for 30 minutes and then re-try
- Chest X-ray – check that the NG tube passes vertically down the oesophagus, in the midline until below the diaphragm. The NG tube must not follow the course of the bronchi. The tip of the NG tube must be visible at least 10cm beyond the gastro-oesophageal junction below the diaphragm

Remove the guidewire from the tube

Tape down tube to secure over the ears and at the nose

Flush with saline

4 To Complete

Thank the patient and tell them that the procedure is finished

Remove PPE and dispose of all waste into appropriate bins

Clean the tray and wash/gel hands

Document the procedure into patient's notes and the pH level

Possible questions you may be asked:
- How often do you check the pH? Check pH and flush tube before every feed
- Care advice: check the surrounding skin, ensure nose remains clean
- How do your remove a NG tube? Use 10ml syringe and inject air down the tube and gently remove

WOUND CARE AND DRESSINGS

Always start with ICE

Assess the wound: site, shape, size, edges/borders, foreign bodies, bleeding/discharge

Assess surrounding area for signs of infection

Dress the wound accordingly

ENT AND SKIN SWABS

Always start with ICE

Ensure to put on appropriate PPE

Check site before swabbing – ear, nose, groin, skin, wound, MRSA screening

Follow instructions

Explain procedure and gain consent

4

Emergency Management

BASIC LIFE SUPPORT – BLS

Unresponsive and not breathing normally

Call 999 and ask for an ambulance

Start 30 chest compressions – 120 compressions per minute (5–6cm depth)

2 rescue breaths (if there is a mouthpiece available) – otherwise leave this part and continue with compressions

30:2 ratio to be carried out if rescue breaths can be given

As soon as AED arrives, switch it on and follow the instructions

IMMEDIATE LIFE SUPPORT - ILS

Unresponsive and not breathing normally

CPR 30:2 - call RESUSCITATION TEAM

Attach DEFIB

Assess rhythm

1. Shockable -VF/Pulseless VT: provide 1 shock and immediately resume CPR for 2 minutes
2. Return of spontaneous circulation: immediate post-cardiac arrest treatment

- Use ABCDE approach
- Aim for SpO2 of 94-98%
- 12-lead ECG
- Treat precipitating cause
- Manage temperature

3 Non-shockable/PEA/Asystole: immediate CPR for 2 minutes

During CPR:

- Ensure high quality chest compressions
- Minimise interruptions to compressions
- Give oxygen
- Use waveform capnography
- Advanced airway in place
- Vascular access (intravenous or intraosseous)
- Give adrenaline every 3-5 minutes
- Give amiodarone after 3 shocks

Treat reversible causes:

REMEMBER YOUR 4Hs and 4Ts

- Hypoxia
- Hypothermia
- Hyperkalaemia/hypokalaemia
- Hypovolaemia
- Toxins
- Tamponade
- Thrombosis – coronary or pulmonary
- Tension pneumothorax

Consider:

- Ultrasound imaging
- Mechanical chest compressions to facilitate transfer/treatment
- Coronary angiography and percutaneous coronary intervention
- Extracorporeal CPR

CHOKING IN ADULT

Assess severity – always start with A–E approach

Check by talking to them, by asking their name, etc. if unable to talk, ask if they can cough, shout for help

If severe airway obstruction with ineffective cough -> unconscious -> start CPR

If severe airway obstruction with ineffective cough -> conscious -> 5 back blows, 5 abdominal thrusts and repeat until airway is clear

If mild airway obstruction with effective cough -> encourage to cough and check for deterioration to ineffective cough or until obstruction is relieved

CHOKING IN CHILD

Depends on child's assess

Always start with A–E approach

Effective cough -> encourage coughing if older child and check for deterioration to ineffective cough or until obstruction is relieved

Ineffective cough -> Unconscious -> 5 rescue breaths and start CPR

Ineffective cough -> Conscious -> 5 back blows, 5 abdominal thrusts (chest for infant) (abdominal for child over >1)

A–E APPROACH

The A–E approach is used for deteriorating and critically ill patients.

Airway, Breathing, Circulation, Disability and Exposure (A–E)

- Before approaching patient always check for personal safety. If available put on apron and gloves and maybe mask.
- 1st observation of patient is a general inspection to see how the patient appears
- If the patient is awake, approach them and ask how they are and check their response
- If there is no response and patient appear unconscious or has collapsed, give them a mild shake and ask again, 'How are you?' If they respond normally, the patient has a patent airway and is breathing (has brain perfusion).
- If the patient only talks in short brief sentences, this may indicate a breathing problem
- If there is no response you may illicit a pain response by doing trapezius pinch
- The first part of 'look, listen and feel' should take only 30 seconds
- If the patient is unconscious, unresponsive and not breathing normally, shout for help and start CPR if patient has no pulse or isn't breathing
- ALWAYS SHOUT FOR HELP, 'Can I get some help here, please!'

General Tips:

- Treat every problem as you find it
- Keep reassessing throughout, after every intervention to check patient's response to treatment
- Always shout for help early and handover using SBA

AIRWAY

- Check if the patient can talk. If so, move on as the airway is patent
- If no, look for signs of airway compromise – cyanosis, use of accessory muscle, abnormal breathing, diminished breath sounds
- Open the mouth and check for obstructing foreign body or secretions
- Open the patient's airway using the head-tilt-chin-lift manoeuvre: place one hand on patient's forehead and under the chin, tilt the forehead back whilst lifting the chin forwards to extend the neck
- Inspect airway for obstruction: if it's visible use a finger sweep or suction to remove it
- If the patient is suspected to have significant trauma with spinal involvement, then perform a jaw thrust instead: identify the angle of the mandible. Use your index and other fingers placed behind the angle of the mandible, apply steady upwards

and forward pressure to lift the mandible. Use your thumbs, slightly open the mouth by doing a downwards displacement of the chin.
- You may need to use airway adjuncts such as oropharyngeal airway (Guedel) or the Nasopharyngeal airway (NPA)
- If the patient loses consciousness and there are no signs of life, call crash team and start CPR immediately.

BREATHING

- Observe patient's respiratory rate; normal rate is between 12-20 per minute
- Check for patient's rise and fall of chest – should take only 10 minutes (look and feel the air on your cheeks at the same time)
- Check oxygen saturation; if below 94% start oxygen 15L via non-rebreather mask
- Check for any cyanosis, obvious shortness of breath, abnormal breathing, wheeze or cough
- Check tracheal position for possible tension pneumothorax
- You can check for chest expansion
- Percuss the chest
- Auscultate for any abnormal, reduced or absent breathing
- You may order investigations such as arterial blood gas (ABG), a chest x-ray, asthma work up

CIRCULATION

- Take the patient's pulse, note the rate, rhythm and volume (normal range between 70-100 beats per minute)
- No pulse: start CPR
- Measure blood pressure
- Signs of hypotension: treat with fluid resuscitation – 500ml bolus of Hartmann's solution or 0.9% sodium chloride initially, if patient at increased risk of fluid overload then give only 250ml boluses, you can repeat this up to 2L, seek senior input at this stage
- Look for obvious pallor, cold peripheries or clammy and sweaty
- Take the capillary refill
- Can assess the JVP
- Auscultate for heart sounds
- Insert a wide bore cannula and take necessary bloods
- Possible blood culture
- 12-lead ECG and continuous cardiac monitoring
- Urine or pregnancy test
- Other culture or swabs
- Fluid output/catheterisation

- Signs of sepsis: manage using FABULOS
- Signs of ACS: manage using MONAC
- Haemorrhage: look for signs of internal or external bleeding

DISABILITY

- Measure level of consciousness using AVPU
- A: alert, is the patient fully alert?
- V: verbal, is the patient making any sounds when you talk to them?
- P: pain, does the patient respond to a pain stimulus i.e., trapezius squeeze or pink or supraorbital pressure?
- U: unresponsive, patient shows no evidence of any eye, voice or motor response to pain
- You can also use the Glasgow Coma Scale (GCS)

Glasgow Coma Scale

Eye, Verbal, Motor – EVM

Eye Opening Response (E)

- Spontaneous – open with blinking at baseline: 4 points
- To verbal stimuli, command, speech: 3 points
- To pain only (not applied to face): 2 points
- No response: 1 point

Verbal Response (V)

- Oriented: 5 points
- Confused conversation, but able to answer questions: 4 points
- Inappropriate words: 3 points
- Incomprehensible speech: 2 points
- No response: 1 point

Motor Response (M)

- Obeys commands for movement: 6 points
- Purposeful movement to painful stimulus: 5 points
- Withdraws in response to pain: 4 points
- Flexion in response to pain (decorticate posturing): 3 points
- Extension response in response to pain (decerebrate posturing): 2 points
- No response: 1 point

Score out of 15, 3 is minimum score

Anything below 8 – suggests severe head injury and requires intubation

- Check pupils
- Drug chart
- VERY IMPORTANT: check capillary blood glucose
- Check ketone levels
- Imaging such as CT/MRI

EXPOSURE

- Inspect patient's skin, colour, temperature, rashes, obvious bleeding
- Swelling to legs
- Obvious wounds
- Treat accordingly

Finish by summarising your findings and your next step, as in senior input/referral, documentation and further investigations and management plans based on your findings.

OXYGEN THERAPY

- Oxygen comes out of a tap which is attached to hospital walls at 100% concentration
- Different devices tolerate different flow rates (0-15l/min). The flow rate can be set on the wall tap.
- The % of oxygen delivery depends on the flow rate and the delivery device
- Intubate if GCS is less than 8
- Aim for oxygen saturations 94-98% in non-COPD patients and 88-92% in COPD patients
- Do an ABG in any patient with oxygen saturations <92%
- Involve ITU if oxygen levels are dropping despite maximal oxygen therapy

Different devices for oxygen delivery

- Nasal cannula: 24-30%, 1-4l can be delivered. Used for non-acute and mildly hypoxic patients
- Mask: 30-40%, 5-10l can be delivered
- Flow rate: 24-60%, used in COPD patients
- Non-rebreather mask: 85-90%, 15l/per minute. Used for acutely ill patients
- Continuous Positive Airway Pressure (CPAP): Used for patients with sleep apnoea, COPD, heart failure
- 100% artificial airway: intubation, in theatre or intensive care unit (ITU)
- Nebuliser can be used in asthmatic patients

INITIAL SEIZURE MANAGEMENT

Use the ABCDE approach

Maintain the airway, give 15l oxygen, gain IV access, ABG/VBG, bloods, ECG, Blood sugar

If the patient has been seizing for 10 minutes, give 4mg IV Lorazepam, if there is no IV access 10-20mg Diazepam PR

If still seizing at 20 minutes, repeat the 4mg Lorazepam dose

30 minutes – IV Phenytoin 18mg/kg

1 Hour/60 minutes – General Anaesthesia in ITU for induced coma

Common causes:

- Metabolic – hypoglycaemia, hyponatraemia, hypocalcaemia
- Eclampsia
- Neurology – epilepsy, brain tumour, meningitis/other infections, trauma to the head/brain
- Febrile convulsions
- Drugs– overdoses, abuse, alcohol intoxication – Thiamine replacement

RECOGNITION AND REVERSAL OF POISONING

Drug	Clinical features	Treatment
Paracetamol	Nausea and vomiting (N&V), abdominal pain – RUQ (24 hrs) jaundice (48 hrs)	• Activated charcoal <1 hr • N-acetylcysteine infusion (NAC) 1st hr – 150mg/kg, 4 hrs – 50mg/kg, 16 hrs- 100mg/kg • Liver transplant occasionally required
Aspirin	Tinnitus, sweating, N&V, abdominal pain, hyperventilation	• Activated charcoal <1 hr • Sodium bicarbonate • Haemodialysis • IV fluids • Check and correct electrolytes
Tricyclics	Drowsiness, confusion, convulsion, coma, dilated pupils, tachycardia, hypotension, increased tone and reflexes	• Activated charcoal <4hrs • Supportive • Sodium bicarbonate
Benzodiazepine	Low GCS	• Supportive – breathing • Do not use Flumazenil unless too much of diazepam was given
Opiates	Reduced GCS, pinpoint pupils, respiratory depression	• Naloxone0.4mg IV • Oxygen and respiratory support

MANAGING ELECTROLYTE DISTURBANCES

HYPOGLYCAEMIA

Signs and symptoms:

- Sweating and clammy
- Dizziness
- Feeling hungry
- Tiredness
- Shaking and trembling
- Tingling lips
- Tachycardia
- Anxious and irritability

Always start with the A–E approach

Alert & orientated and blood glucose concentration is less than 4mmol/l with or without symptoms:

Provide them with 15-20g oral carbohydrate

Rapid acting – sugary drink – 3-4 heaped teaspoons of sugar dissolved in water or 150-200 ml of pure fruit juice.

If necessary can repeat this treatment every 10 -15 minutes, up to 3 times. Once patient has recovered and the blood sugar concentration is over 4 mmol/l then provide a long-acting carbohydrate such as one slice of bread, 200 ml of milk or 2 biscuits.

Drowsy/confused but swallow is intact:

Provide them with buccal treatment

Hypo stop/Glucose – Glucogel is usually used

Can consider IV access at this point

If the hypoglycaemia does not respond to above treatments after 3 cycles and it's over 40 minutes

Or the patient is unconscious or concerned re swallow:

IV dextrose

100ml 20% dextrose

If they are deteriorating and there is no IV access:

1mg glucagon IM/SC

HYPERGLYCAEMIA

Signs and symptoms:
- Increased thirst and dry mouth
- Blurred vision
- Abdominal pain
- Unintentional weight loss
- Polyuria
- Fatigue
- N&V

Suspected diabetes ketoacidosis (DKA):

- Acidosis (pH <7.3 +\- HCO3 <15mM)
- Hyperglycaemia 11.1mmol/l or > or known DM
- Ketonaemia 2+ or > on dipstick/point of care testing

How to manage DKA:

- REMEMBER IT'S FLUIDS FIRST
- 0.9% normal saline infusion (Systolic BP 90<) 1l over 1hr
- 1l over next 2hr, 1l/2hr, 1l/4hr, 1l/4hr, 1l/6hr
- Switch to 10% dextrose 1l/8h when glucose 14mmol/l
- 0.1/kg/h Actrapid Insulin (approx. 50 units)
- Potassium replacement may be needed if in the 2nd bag of fluids:

If potassium is 5.5mM – normal

If between 3.5-5.5mM – will require 40mM

If less than 3.5mM – will require a consultant/senior review

Electrolyte	Causes	Investigations	Management
Hypokalaemia	Increased renal excretion via diuretics, steroids, Cushing's or Conn's syndrome. Intestinal loss via V&D, increased cellular uptake – salbutamol, insulin and alkalosis	Potassium levels	- >2.5mmol/l: Sando K 2 tablets TDS or add 20-40mmol/l potassium chloride to IV fluids - <2.5mmol/l: 40mmol/l potassium chloride in 1l 0.9& saline over 6 hours - Never give >10mmol/hr unless in ITU or senior level - Treat cause
Hyperkalaemia	Reduced renal excretion: acute or chronic kidney injury, drugs i.e. ACEi NSAIDS, Addison's Disease. Excess potassium load, acidosis.	Potassium levels	- ECG and cardiac monitoring- low/flat P waves, wide bizarre QRS, tall tented/peaky T waves - Calcium gluconate 10ml 10% IV over 5 minutes - Actrapid insulin 10 units - Calcium resonium - Treat cause
Hyponatraemia	Hypovolaemia, euvolemia, hypervolaemia	Plasma osmolality, urinary sodium and osmolality	Treat the cause Sodium correction
Hypernatraemia	Iatrogenic – hypervolaemia – iv fluids	Urine and serum osmolality	Treat the cause Sodium correction

FLUID RESUSCITATION

When may you need a fluid resuscitation?

Causes of shock:

- Sepsis
- Burns
- Haemorrhage
- Fluid loss via diarrhoea and vomiting

Initial Assessment
Always start with AE approach

Clinical observations should all be done

Red flag for hypovolaemia -> hypotension + tachycardia + reduced urine output

Patient will require a wide bore cannula and take all urgent bloods including for clotting and transfusion – crossmatch for 4 units

Fluid Resus

Give a fluid bolus of 500 ml crystalloid solution via IV such as NaCl 0.9%/Hartmann's solution within 15 minutes

Reassess again using the A-E approach

If they are still showing signs of hypovolemia -> give them a further 250ml – 500ml of crystalloid solution

Again reassess

Repeat this until you have reached 2l, if the patient hasn't improved by then, urgent senior review is required

If the patient is at risk of fluid overload due to liver failure, heart failure or kidney disease, then give fluid boluses with caution by starting with 250 ml of fluid initially and seek early senior review

SEPSIS MANAGEMENT

Sepsis is a life-threatening organ dysfunction, usually starts with localised infection such as pneumonia, skin wounds, through invasive lines, cholecystitis, pancreatitis and more commonly urine infections.

It is described as an inflammatory response initiated by endotoxin derived from gram negative bacteria.

Risk levels are low – high

Low-moderate risk

- Respiratory rate: 21-24 breaths per minute
- SBP: 91-100mmHg
- HR: 91-130 bpm
- Temperature: <36 degrees

High risk

- Respiratory rate: 25 or more breaths per minute
- SBP: 90/40 mmHg
- HR: >130 bpm
- Temperature: >36 degrees

Septic shock: sepsis hypotension that does not respond to adequate fluid resuscitation and/or evidence of end-organ dysfunction or failure. (SBP <90/40)

Scoring systems

- Quick SOFA
- SIRS criteria:

Systemic Inflammatory Response Syndrome

Two or more of the following:

- Temperature >38°C or <36°C
- Tachycardia: >90 beats per minute
- Tachypnoea: >20 breaths per minute) or PCO2 <4.3kPa
- WCC >12 or <4 (or >10% immature (band) forms)
- Rash/mottled skin
- Unwell
- Altered mental state
- Nausea and vomiting

Risk factors:

- Very elderly
- Very young
- Immunocompromised patients i.e. chemotherapy patients, diabetes, steroid use, AIDS
- Pregnant
- Recent surgery

Management of sepsis

Remember: take 3 and give 3

Take:

- Take blood cultures, take lactate – ABG, take urine output
- Give IV antibiotics, give oxygen, give IV fluids

Always start with A-E approach and do all your necessary clinical observations, treat each finding as you go along and keep reassessing.

This can help to remember:

F Fluids – 500ml of 0.9 % saline over 15 minutes
A Antibiotics – Broad spectrum antibiotics – Benzylpenicillin, Cefotaxime, Amoxicillin, Gentamicin
B Blood cultures and normal bloods
U Urine output/catheter – monitor every 30 minutes
L Lactate
O Oxygen – 15l via non rebreather mask
S Sixty minutes (within the golden 60 minutes)

Review the patient after 1 hour

NOSE BLEED (EPISTAXIS) MANAGEMENT

Causes of epistaxis:

- Primary/idiopathic (80-85%) or secondary
- Local – trauma (fracture, nose picking, foreign body, post-operative), infections (rhinitis, sinusitis), neoplasms (malignancy, juvenile angiofibroma, inverted papilloma)
- Systemic – drugs (anticoagulants, cocaine), haematological conditions (haemophilia , leukaemia), hypertension

Location of bleeds

- Anterior bleed (most common) usually from the Little's Area (Kiesselbach's plexus) or anterior-inferior septum, internal carotid artery to anterior ethmoidal, external carotid artery to superior labial
- Posterior bleed (less common) from Woodruff's plexus

Management

After taking a good history:

Start with A-E approach if patient is acutely unwell

Ensure airway is not compromised by the bleeding and the patient is not in shock

Resuscitate with IV access and fluids if required

1st aid management: sit patient forward, pinch the soft fleshy part of the nose, you can place ice on forehead or back of the neck. Instruct to spit blood into a vomit bowl to avoid nausea and vomiting.

If bleed continues more than 20 minutes, you can use Co-phenylcaine local anaesthetic spray which is a decongestant and vasoconstrictor

You may need to use silver nitrate to cauterise the vessel causing the bleed

If bleeding continues, anterior packing and admission maybe required

Always assess with A-E approach

Will depend on severity

REFERENCE LIST

While compiling this book the author has drawn on the public sources below for guidance.

A CODE OF PRACTICE FOR THE DIAGNOSIS AND CONFIRMATION OF DEATH. (n.d.). [online]. Available at: https://aomrc.org.uk/wp-content/uploads/2016/04/Code_Practice_Confirmation_Diagnosis_Death_1008-4.pdf.

Ahmed, S.M., Lemkau, J.P. and Birt, S.L. (2002). Toward Sensitive Treatment of Obese Patients in Primary Care. *Family Practice Management*, [online] 9(1), p.25. Available at: https://www.aafp.org/fpm/2002/0100/p25.html [Accessed 9 Jul. 2021].

Amerson, J.R. (1990). *Inguinal Canal and Hernia Examination*. 3rd ed. [online] PubMed. Available at: https://www.ncbi.nlm.nih.gov/books/NBK423/.

Baile, W.F. (2000). SPIKES--A Six-Step Protocol for Delivering Bad News: Application to the Patient with Cancer. *The Oncologist*, [online] 5(4), pp.302–311. Available at: http://theoncologist.alphamedpress.org/content/5/4/302.long.

Bharati, K. and Munakomi, S. (2020). *Intramuscular Injection*. [online] PubMed. Available at: https://www.ncbi.nlm.nih.gov/books/NBK556121/.

Brief Interventions for Smoking Cessation - HSE.ie (2016). *Brief Interventions for Smoking Cessation - HSE.ie*. [online] HSE.ie. Available at: https://www.hse.ie/eng/about/who/tobaccocontrol/intervention/.

Church, D.J., Krumme, J. and Kotwal, S. (2017). Evaluating Soft-Tissue Lumps and Bumps. *Missouri Medicine*, [online] 114(4), pp.289–294. Available at: https://www.ncbi.nlm.nih.gov/pmc/articles/PMC6140092/.

Clare, S. and Rowley, S. (2017). *Implementing the Aseptic Non Touch Technique (ANTT®) clinical practice framework for aseptic technique: a pragmatic evaluation using a mixed methods approach in two London hospitals*. [online] Europe PMC. Available at: https://europepmc.org/article/PMC/PMC5753945.

Cook, F., Lavery, I. and McGibbon, A. (2009). *REGISTERED NURSE*. [online] NHS Lothian. Available at: file:///C:/Users/amz78/AppData/Local/Microsoft/Windows/INetCache/IE/9HRO0S76/Nurse%20Verification%20of%20Expected%20Death%20May%202009.pdf.

DeVrieze, B.W. and Giwa, A.O. (2020). *Peak Flow Rate Measurement*. [online] PubMed. Available at: https://www.ncbi.nlm.nih.gov/books/NBK459325/.

Dr Colin Tidy (2016). *Cardiovascular Risk Assessment*. [online] Patient.info. Available at: https://patient.info/doctor/cardiovascular-risk-assessment.

Dr Supreet Sidhu (2017a). *Breaking Bad News*. [online] Geeky Medics. Available at: https://geekymedics.com/breaking-bad-news/.

Dr Supreet Sidhu (2017b). *Dealing with Angry Patients and Relatives*. [online] Geeky Medics. Available at: https://geekymedics.com/dealing-angry-patients-relatives/.

Education, M. and Hiramatsu, S. (2019). *OSCE course*. [Face to face, powerpoint presentations and notes].

Ernst, D.J. and Ernst, C. (2002). Phlebotomy tools of the trade. *Home Healthcare Nurse*, [online] 20(3), pp.151–153. Available at: https://pubmed.ncbi.nlm.nih.gov/11984175/ [Accessed 9 Jul. 2021].

Ferguson, C.M. (2011). *Inspection, Auscultation, Palpation, and Percussion of the Abdomen*. [online] Nih.gov. Available at: https://www.ncbi.nlm.nih.gov/books/NBK420/.

General practice - A safe place. (n.d.). [online]. Available at: https://www.racgp.org.au/download/Documents/PracticeSupport/17185-general-practice-a-safe-place.pdf.

Gibbs, H.R. (1990). *History of Cardiovascular Disease*. 3rd ed. [online] PubMed. Available at: https://www.ncbi.nlm.nih.gov/books/NBK246/.

Gregory, J., Wood, S. and Proske, U. (2001). An investigation into mechanisms of reflex reinforcement by the Jendrassik manoeuvre. *Experimental Brain Research*, [online] 138(3), pp.366–374. Available at: http://plaza.ufl.edu/cphadke/PDF's/E/Gregory2001%20Jendrassik-H-reflex.pdf [Accessed 19 Nov. 2019].

Gudlavalleti, A. and Tenny, S. (2021). *Cerebellar Neurological Signs*. [online] PubMed. Available at: https://www.ncbi.nlm.nih.gov/books/NBK556080/.

healthservice.hse.ie. (n.d.). *ONMSD*. [online] Available at: http://www.hse.ie/eng/about/who/onmsd [Accessed 9 Jul. 2021].

Henderson, J.A. and Ferguson, T. (2020). *Breast Examination Techniques*. [online] PubMed. Available at: https://www.ncbi.nlm.nih.gov/books/NBK459179/.

http://typework.com (2015). *ERC Guidelines 2015 have arrived, download them now!* [online] Guidelines. Available at: https://cprguidelines.eu/.

Hutchison, A.S., Ralston, S.H., Dryburgh, F.J., Small, M. and Fogelman, I. (1983). Too much heparin: possible source of error in blood gas analysis. *British Medical Journal (Clinical research ed.)*, [online] 287(6399), pp.1131–1132. Available at: https://www.ncbi.nlm.nih.gov/pmc/articles/PMC1549341/ [Accessed 9 Jul. 2021].

Ialongo, C. and Bernardini, S. (2016). Phlebotomy, a bridge between laboratory and patient. *Biochemia Medica*, [online] pp.17–33. Available at: https://www.ncbi.nlm.nih.gov/pmc/articles/PMC4783087/.

Implementation advice 2007 NICE clinical guideline 50. (n.d.). [online] . Available at: https://www.nice.org.uk/guidance/cg50/resources/implementation-advice-pdf-433575469.

Jakes, A.D., Whybrow, R., Spencer, C. and Chappell, L.C. (2018). Reduced fetal movements. *BMJ*, [online] p.k570. Available at: https://www.bmj.com/content/360/bmj.k570 [Accessed 15 Oct. 2019].

Kreugel, G., Beijer, H., Kerstens, M., ter Maaten, J., Sluiter, W. and Boot, B. (2007). Influence of needle size for subcutaneous insulin administration on metabolic control and patient acceptance. *European Diabetes Nursing*, 4(2), pp.51–55.

Krogsbøll, L.T. (2014). Guidelines for screening with urinary dipsticks differ substantially--a systematic review. *Danish Medical Journal*, [online] 61(2), p.A4781. Available at: https://pubmed.ncbi.nlm.nih.gov/24495888/ [Accessed 9 Jul. 2021].

Krogsbøll, L.T., Jørgensen, K.J. and Gøtzsche, P.C. (2015). Screening with urinary dipsticks for reducing morbidity and mortality. *Cochrane Database of Systematic Reviews*.

Lee, J.W. (2010). Fluid and Electrolyte Disturbances in Critically Ill Patients. *Electrolytes & Blood Pressure*, 8(2), p.72.

Lee, S.-H. (2014). Colonoscopy procedural skills and training for new beginners. *World Journal of Gastroenterology*, 20(45), p.16984.

Lee, S.-H., Park, Y.-K., Cho, S.-M., Kang, J.-K. and Lee, D.-J. (2015). Technical skills and training of upper gastrointestinal endoscopy for new beginners. *World Journal of Gastroenterology : WJG*, [online] 21(3), pp.759–785. Available at: https://www.ncbi.nlm.nih.gov/pmc/articles/PMC4299329/.

Martin, D.C. (2016). *The Mental Status Examination*. [online] Nih.gov. Available at: https://www.ncbi.nlm.nih.gov/books/NBK320/.

McFarlane, M.J. (1990). *The Rectal Examination*. 3rd ed. [online] PubMed. Available at: https://www.ncbi.nlm.nih.gov/books/NBK424/.

Meek, S. (2002). ABC of clinical electrocardiography: Introduction. I---Leads, rate, rhythm, and cardiac axis. *BMJ*, [online] 324(7334), pp.415–418. Available at: https://www.ncbi.nlm.nih.gov/pmc/articles/PMC1122339/.

Myers, K., Mcrobbie, H., West, O. and Hajek, P. (2012). *Smoking cessation in Secondary Care Review 3 (Component 1) Smoking cessation interventions in acute and maternity services: Review of Barriers and Facilitators Report to National Institute for Health and Clinical Excellence Final Draft*. [online] . Available at: https://www.nice.org.uk/guidance/ph48/evidence/review-3-barriers-facilitators-for-smoking-cessation-interventions-in-acute-and-maternity-services-pdf-430361391.

National Institute for Health and Care Excellence (2019). *Oxygen*. [online] NICE. Available at: https://bnf.nice.org.uk/treatment-summary/oxygen.html.

NICE (2014). *Overview | Cardiovascular disease: risk assessment and reduction, including lipid modification | Guidance | NICE*. [online] Nice.org.uk. Available at: https://www.nice.org.uk/guidance/cg181.

NICE (2017). *Recommendations | Asthma: diagnosis, monitoring and chronic asthma management | Guidance | NICE*. [online] Nice.org.uk. Available at: https://www.nice.org.uk/guidance/ng80/chapter/Recommendations.

NICE (2020). *National Early Warning Score systems that alert to deteriorating adult patients in hospital*. [online]. Available at:https://www.nice.org.uk/advice/mib205/resources/national-early-warning-score-systems-that-alert-to-deteriorating-adult-patients-in-hospital-pdf-2285965392761797.

NICE. (n.d.). *CKS is only available in the UK*. [online] Available at: https://cks.nice.org.uk/topics/meningitis-bacterial-meningitis-meningococcal-disease/diagnosis/assessing-the-rash/.

NICE. (n.d.). *CKS is only available in the UK*. [online] Available at: https://cks.nice.org.uk/topics/chest-infections-adult/diagnosis/assessment/.

NICE. (n.d.). *CKS is only available in the UK*. [online] Available at: https://cks.nice.org.uk/topics/carpal-tunnel-syndrome/diagnosis/diagnosis/.

NICE. (n.d.). *CKS is only available in the UK*. [online] Available at: https://cks.nice.org.uk/topics/back-pain-low-without-radiculopathy/diagnosis/diagnosis/.

NICE. (n.d.). *CKS is only available in the UK*. [online] Available at: https://cks.nice.org.uk/topics/shoulder-pain/diagnosis/diagnosis/.

NICE. (n.d.). *CKS is only available in the UK*. [online] Available at: https://cks.nice.org.uk/topics/greater-trochanteric-pain-syndrome/diagnosis/differential-diagnosis/ [Accessed 9 Jul. 2021].

NICE. (n.d.). *CKS is only available in the UK*. [online] Available at: https://cks.nice.org.uk/topics/knee-pain-assessment/diagnosis/examination/.

NICE. (n.d.). *CKS is only available in the UK*. [online] Available at: https://cks.nice.org.uk/topics/vaginal-discharge/diagnosis/examination-investigations/ [Accessed 9 Jul. 2021].

NICE. (n.d.). *CKS is only available in the UK.* [online] Available at: https://cks.nice.org.uk/topics/obesity/diagnosis/identification-classification/.
NICE. (n.d.). *CKS is only available in the UK.* [online] Available at: https://cks.nice.org.uk/topics/cardiac-arrest-out-of-hospital-care/management/basic-life-support-adult/.
NICE. (n.d.). *CKS is only available in the UK.* [online] Available at: https://cks.nice.org.uk/topics/lacerations/management/laceration-low-infection-risk/.
Nice.org.uk. (2015a). *Evidence context | Wound care products | Advice | NICE.* [online] Available at: https://www.nice.org.uk/advice/ktt14/chapter/Evidence-context.
Nice.org.uk. (2015b). *Recommendations | Diabetic foot problems: prevention and management | Guidance | NICE.* [online] Available at: https://www.nice.org.uk/guidance/ng19/chapter/Recommendations#assessing-the-risk-of-developing-a-diabetic-foot-problem.
NT Contributor (2009). *Reducing the risk of infection with indwelling urethral catheters | Nursing Times.* [online] Nursing Times. Available at: https://www.nursingtimes.net/clinical-archive/infection-control/reducing-the-risk-of-infection-with-indwelling-urethral-catheters-17-09-2009/.
Office of the Nursing and Midwifery Servics Director. Health Service Executive (2017). *Guiding Framework for the Education, Training and.* [online] Available at: http://hdl.handle.net/10147/622531.
Okhunov, Z., Hruby, G.W., Mirabile, G., Marruffo, F., Lehman, D.S., Benson, M.C., Gupta, M. and Landman, J. (2009). Prospective Comparison of Flexible Fiberoptic and Digital Cystoscopes. *Urology*, 74(2), pp.427–430.
Papagrigoriadis, S. (2004). Evaluation of flexible sigmoidoscopy as an investigation for "left sided" colorectal symptoms. *Postgraduate Medical Journal*, 80(940), pp.104–106.
Paradis, T.J., Dixon, J. and Tieu, B.H. (2016). The role of bronchoscopy in the diagnosis of airway disease. *Journal of Thoracic Disease*, [online] 8(12), pp.3826–3837. Available at: https://www.ncbi.nlm.nih.gov/pmc/articles/PMC5227188/.
patient.info. (n.d.). *Neurological Examination of the Upper Limbs. Information.* [online] Available at: https://patient.info/doctor/neurological-examination-of-the-upper-limbs.
Pope, L.E.R. and Hobbs, C.G.L. (2005). Epistaxis: an update on current management. *Postgraduate Medical Journal*, [online] 81(955), pp.309–314. Available at: https://pmj.bmj.com/content/81/955/309.long [Accessed 17 May 2020].
Public Health England (2017). *Cost of smoking to the NHS in England: 2015.* [online] GOV.UK. Available at: https://www.gov.uk/government/publications/cost-of-smoking-to-the-nhs-in-england-2015/cost-of-smoking-to-the-nhs-in-england-2015.
Puri, S., Paul, G. and Sood, P. (2010). Interpretation of arterial blood gas. *Indian Journal of Critical Care Medicine*, [online] 14(2), pp.57–64. Available at: https://www.ncbi.nlm.nih.gov/pmc/articles/PMC2936733/.
Reddel, H.K., Taylor, D.R., Bateman, E.D., Boulet, L.-P., Boushey, H.A., Busse, W.W., Casale, T.B., Chanez, P., Enright, P.L., Gibson, P.G., de Jongste, J.C., Kerstjens, H.A.M., Lazarus, S.C., Levy, M.L., O'Byrne, P.M., Partridge, M.R., Pavord, I.D., Sears, M.R., Sterk, P.J. and Stoloff, S.W. (2009). An Official American Thoracic Society/European Respiratory Society Statement: Asthma Control and Exacerbations. *American Journal of Respiratory and Critical Care Medicine*, 180(1), pp.59–99.
Rivers, E., Nguyen, B., Havstad, S., Ressler, J., Muzzin, A., Knoblich, B., Peterson, E. and Tomlanovich, M. (2001). Early Goal-Directed Therapy in the Treatment of Severe Sepsis and Septic Shock. *New England Journal of Medicine*, [online] 345(19), pp.1368–1377. Available at: https://www.nejm.org/doi/full/10.1056/NEJMoa010307.
Rundo, F., Conoci, S., Ortis, A. and Battiato, S. (2018). An Advanced Bio-Inspired PhotoPlethysmoGraphy (PPG) and ECG Pattern Recognition System for Medical Assessment. *Sensors*, 18(2), p.405.
Sattar, Y. and Chhabra, L. (2020). *Electrocardiogram.* [online] PubMed. Available at: https://www.ncbi.nlm.nih.gov/books/NBK549803/.
Seizure prognosis of patients with low-grade tumors. (2012). *Seizure*, [online] 21(7), pp.540–545. Available at: https://www.sciencedirect.com/science/article/pii/S1059131112001446 [Accessed 9 Jul. 2021].
Shaw, H. (2015). Intramuscular injection. *Nursing Standard*, 30(6), pp.61–62.
Sigmon, D. and An, J. (2021). Nasogastric Tube. *StatPearls.* [online] Available at: https://www.statpearls.com/ArticleLibrary/viewarticle/25555.
simpleosce.com. (n.d.). *Peak expiratory flow station - OSCE.* [online] Available at: https://simpleosce.com/procedures/peak-expiratory-flow.php [Accessed 9 Jul. 2021].
SMOKING CESSATION IN PRIMARY CARE A CROSS-SECTIONAL SURVEY OF PRIMARY CARE HEALTH PRACTITIONERS IN THE UK AND THE USE OF VERY BRIEF ADVICE EXECUTIVE SUMMARY BACKGROUND. (2019). [online] . Available at: https://www.cancerresearchuk.org/sites/default/files/tobacco_pc_report_to_publish_-_exec_summary.pdf [Accessed 9 Jul. 2021].

Suspected neurological conditions: recognition and referral NICE guideline. (2019). [online] . Available at: https://www.nice.org.uk/guidance/ng127/resources/suspected-neurological-conditions-recognition-and-referral-pdf-66141663923653.

ten Broek, R.P.G., Krielen, P., Di Saverio, S., Coccolini, F., Biffl, W.L., Ansaloni, L., Velmahos, G.C., Sartelli, M., Fraga, G.P., Kelly, M.D., Moore, F.A., Peitzman, A.B., Leppaniemi, A., Moore, E.E., Jeekel, J., Kluger, Y., Sugrue, M., Balogh, Z.J., Bendinelli, C. and Civil, I. (2018). Bologna guidelines for diagnosis and management of adhesive small bowel obstruction (ASBO): 2017 update of the evidence-based guidelines from the world society of emergency surgery ASBO working group. *World Journal of Emergency Surgery*, 13(1).

The epidemiology and impact of gambling disorder and other gambling-related harm Enhancing public health actions through partnerships and collaboration. (2017). [online] . Available at: https://www.who.int/docs/default-source/substance-use/the-epidemiology-and-impact-of-gambling-disorder-and-other-gambling-relate-harm.pdf?sfvrsn=5901c849_2.

Tidy, C. (2014). *Examination of the Cranial Nerves. Cranial Information. Patient.* [online] patient.info. Available at: https://patient.info/doctor/examination-of-the-cranial-nerves.

Ubbink, D.T., Brölmann, F.E., Go, P.M.N.Y.H. and Vermeulen, H. (2015). Evidence-Based Care of Acute Wounds: A Perspective. *Advances in Wound Care*, [online] 4(5), pp.286–294. Available at: https://www.ncbi.nlm.nih.gov/pmc/articles/PMC4432965/ [Accessed 6 May 2019].

updated:January 11, C.R. giving-Last and 2021 (n.d.). *Explaining a Diagnosis of Diabetes - OSCE Guide | Geeky Medics.* [online] Available at: https://geekymedics.com/explaining-a-diagnosis-of-diabetes-osce-guide/ [Accessed 9 Jul. 2021].

Usach, I., Martinez, R., Festini, T. and Peris, J.-E. (2019). Subcutaneous Injection of Drugs: Literature Review of Factors Influencing Pain Sensation at the Injection Site. *Advances in Therapy*, 36(11), pp.2986–2996.

WEBB, S.S., PLANA, M.N., ZAMORA, J., AHMAD, A., EARLEY, B., MACARTHUR, C. and KHAN, K.S. (2011). Abdominal palpation to determine fetal position at labor onset: a test accuracy study. *Acta Obstetricia et Gynecologica Scandinavica*, 90(11), pp.1259–1266.

www.nice.org.uk. (2012). *Guidance | Epilepsies: diagnosis and management | Guidance | NICE.* [online] Available at: https://www.nice.org.uk/guidance/cg137/chapter/1-Guidance#diagnosis-2.

www.nice.org.uk. (n.d.). *Recommendations | Hearing loss in adults: assessment and management | Guidance | NICE.* [online] Available at: https://www.nice.org.uk/guidance/ng98/chapter/Recommendations#assessment-and-referral.

www.nice.org.uk. (n.d.). *Recommendations | Peripheral arterial disease: diagnosis and management | Guidance | NICE.* [online] Available at: https://www.nice.org.uk/guidance/cg147/chapter/Recommendations#diagnosis.

www.nice.org.uk. (n.d.). *Recommendations | Urinary tract infection (catheter-associated): antimicrobial prescribing | Guidance | NICE.* [online] Available at: https://www.nice.org.uk/guidance/ng113/chapter/Recommendations.

www.nice.org.uk. (n.d.). *Skin and soft tissue | Information for the public | Suspected cancer: recognition and referral | Guidance | NICE.* [online] Available at: https://www.nice.org.uk/guidance/ng12/ifp/chapter/Skin-and-soft-tissue [Accessed 9 Jul. 2021].

www.uptodate.com. (n.d.). *UpToDate.* [online] Available at: https://www.uptodate.com/contents/search?search=behavioral-approaches-to-smokingcessation&sp=0&searchType=PLAIN_TEXT&source=USER_INPUT&searchControl=TOP_PULLDOWN&searchOffset=1&autoComplete=false&language=&max=0&index=&autoCompleteTerm=&rawSentence= [Accessed 9 Jul. 2021].

YEH, J.M., HUR, C., WARD, Z. and SCHRAG, D. (2015). *Europe PMC.* [online] europepmc.org. Available at: https://europepmc.org/article/PMC/4573370#free-full-text [Accessed 9 Jul. 2021].